A Hazelden Pocket Health Guide

High Blood Pressure

Practical, Medical, and Spiritual Guidelines for Daily Living with Hypertension

MARK JENKINS

Foreword by Robert E. Larsen, M.D.

1949-1999
HAZELDEN

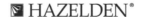

HAZELDEN®

INFORMATION & EDUCATIONAL SERVICES

Hazelden
Center City, Minnesota 55012-0176

1-800-328-0094
1-651-213-4590 (Fax)
www.hazelden.org

Library of Congress Cataloging-in-Publication Data

Jenkins, Mark, 1962–
    High blood pressure : practical, medical, and spiritual guidelines
  for daily living with hypertension / Mark Jenkins ; foreword by
  Robert E. Larsen.
        p.   cm. — (A Hazelden pocket health guide)
    Includes bibliographical references and index.
    ISBN 1-56838-351-7
    1. Hypertension Popular works. 2. Hypertension—Psychosomatic
  aspects. 3. Twelve-step programs. 4. Adjustment (Psychology)
  I. Title. II. Series.
  RC685.H8J46   1999
  616.1'32—dc21   99-32798
                                                                 CIP

03 02 01 00 99   6 5 4 3 2 1

Editor's note
The excerpt from the book *Alcoholics Anonymous,* pages 83–84, and the
Twelve Steps are reprinted /adapted with permission of Alcoholics Anonymous
World Services, Inc. Permission to reprint pages 83–84 and the Twelve Steps
does not mean that AA has reviewed or approved the contents of this publication, or that AA necessarily agrees with the views expressed herein. AA is a
program of recovery from alcoholism *only*—use of pages 83–84 and the Twelve
Steps in connection with programs and activities which are patterned after AA,
but which address other problems, or in any other non-AA context, does not
imply otherwise.

Cover design by David Spohn
Interior design by Donna Burch
Typesetting by Stanton Publication Services, Inc.

High Blood Pressure

Contents

Foreword by Robert E. Larsen, M.D.   vii

Preface   xi

Introduction—
    Spirituality: The Strongest Medicine of All?   xv

Chapter 1: Hypertension Essentials   1
    What Is Blood Pressure and What Happens
    When It Is High?; Causes of Hypertension;
    Who Is Likely to Develop High Blood Pressure?;
    Symptoms of Hypertension; Understanding Blood
    Pressure Readings; Diagnosing Hypertension;
    Hypertension: Incurable but Controllable;
    Hypertension: The Mind-Body Connection;
    Effects of High Blood Pressure

Chapter 2: A Spiritual Program to
    Help Manage Hypertension   21
    Twelve Step How-To; Step One: The Foundation
    of Recovery; Step Two: A Promise of Hope;
    Step Three: Turning It Over; Step Four: Knowing
    Yourself; Step Five: Telling My Story; Step Six:
    Ready, Willing, and Able; Step Seven: Being
    Changed; Step Eight: Preparing for Change;
    Step Nine: Facing the Past; Step Ten: Maintaining
    Our New Lives; Step Eleven: Partnership with a
    Higher Power; Step Twelve: Carrying the Message;
    Step by Step

Chapter 3: Containing Your Hypertension   53

Avoiding the Easy Path; Behavior Modification;
Medication for Hypertension; Commitment to a
Spiritual Program

Chapter 4: Women and Hypertension   91

The Age Factor; Women, Race, and Hypertension;
Pregnancy and Hypertension; Effects of Birth
Control Medication

Chapter 5: Exercise to Control
        High Blood Pressure   99

What Is Fitness?; Fitness Fundamentals;
Maintaining Fitness and Lowered Blood Pressure;
Exercising for Weight Loss; The Importance of
Flexibility Exercises and Strength Training

Chapter 6: Complementary and Alternative
        Treatments for Hypertension   117

How to Find Out More about Complementary
and Alternative Treatments for Hypertension;
How to Find a Practitioner in Your Area; What to
Consider When Choosing an Alternative Health
Therapy or Practitioner; Specific Alternative/
Complementary Treatments for Hypertension

Appendix   131

Index   135

About the Author   149

Foreword

For the past sixty years, millions of addicts and alcoholics have stopped using drugs and found new, rewarding lives by following the spiritual principles outlined in Twelve Step programs such as Alcoholics Anonymous. From a medical perspective, it is not unreasonable to say that Twelve Step programs constitute the gold standard of treatment for the chronic disease of chemical dependency. These programs have been so successful that they are now used to deal with other challenges of a chronic nature, such as overeating, sexual compulsion, gambling, and depression.

The Hazelden Pocket Health Guide series is designed to help patients cope with chronic diseases, specifically, diseases that may be the result of an addiction. These long-term, potentially debilitating illnesses include chronic obstructive pulmonary disease (COPD), hypertension, and liver disease. This series can help patients use the same spiritual principles that have enabled so many chemically dependent people to lead full and satisfying lives.

Spirituality and acceptance are powerful tools patients and health care professionals can apply to help deal with disease. In thirty years of medical practice, I have seen many patients with chronic disease who, despite the best physicians and hospitals, have done poorly. Sometimes this was due to the severity of the disease process, but often, the patient's inability to accept the disease and its consequences was significant. Denial is a common problem in chemically dependent people, but chemical dependency is by no means the only disease in which it plays a major role in the outcome. Denial is common to *every* chronic disease known to medical science. If not dealt with effectively, it is a major stumbling block to effective treatment.

Despite significant advances in treating diabetes, for instance, at least half of all diabetics fail to follow their diets or to take their medications properly. Many of these patients suffer amputations, kidney failure and dialysis, heart attacks, and blindness partly due to their disease but mostly due to the denial that blinds them to effective treatment of the disease.

Denial and chronic disease can be dealt with by using spiritual principles. Spirituality is not religion, although some people achieve it in traditional religious communities. Spirituality is the concept that each of us has a Higher Power that can help us cope with life. For many this is the traditional God, while for others it may be nature, the recovering community, or a set of guiding principles. Each person has his or her own concept of a Higher Power. Spirituality is not a particular religious dogma but rather a concept that allows people to feel good about how they live their lives.

Bill Wilson, the cofounder of Alcoholics Anonymous, described the concept of spirituality as the concept that we can do together what we could not do alone. Spirituality is about community and being a part of a greater whole. Spirituality is we *not* me.

Hypertension

Hypertension, the silent killer. Despite large public health efforts that have seen the death rate from heart disease decrease significantly, hypertension is still a major cause of death in the United States. Unfortunately, no symptoms are associated with this condition until major damage is done to vital organs including the heart, brain, and kidneys. This leads many people with hypertension to ignore their condition. The result is permanent damage that leads to extreme illness or death.

Even with excellent health care facilities and a strong public health effort, only an estimated 25 percent of people with hypertension seek treatment. Furthermore, many of those who do seek treatment fail to take their medications regularly and do not make the lifestyle changes necessary to treat their condition adequately.

Much of this is due to denial. Because many patients have no symptoms, they refuse to believe they are ill. Others may acknowledge their illness but fail to treat it properly, believing that they will have time, in the future, to get serious about treatment. They may think, Why should I put up with side effects of medication when I feel fine? In short, many fail to accept their condition and take the necessary steps to ensure the proper treatment of this life-threatening disease. Applying the principles found in this book will help the patient with hypertension to better accept and treat this silent killer.

Robert E. Larsen, M.D.
Coordinator, Health Care Professionals Program
Hazelden Foundation

Preface

I owe my life to a spiritual program of recovery. My journey started when I joined the recovery community. By following the Twelve Steps of Alcoholics Anonymous (the basis of all Twelve Step programs), I found a new life. My career was rebuilt, my relationships with others mended, my self-esteem restored.

A natural-born cynic, I was at first astounded when so many of "the Promises" I had been told about came true, and in such short order (see pages xix–xx for more on the Promises). Even by then, I had learned not to question but to simply accept such blessings as part of my continuing journey.

As a medical writer with several books to my credit, I began to postulate that this spiritual program of recovery would be a revelation to people with chronic illnesses. After all, the Twelve Steps are a universal plan for living well. Countless groups apply the Twelve Steps to their addictions and conditions—including Emotions Anonymous, Debtors Anonymous, Gamblers Anonymous, and, the grandparent of them all, Alcoholics Anonymous. And so I set about writing a book that offers a spiritual program of recovery from chronic illness.

Probably no one needs a guide to living well more

than people who suffer from long-term medical conditions. Chronic illness affects more than ninety million Americans and, according to the American Medical Association, is the nation's foremost health concern. Chronic illness can lead to feelings of anger, isolation and loneliness, financial difficulties, compromised personal relationships, and trouble at work. The emotional consequences of a chronic illness are especially profound when the condition is caused by a dependency on a mood-altering substance such as nicotine or alcohol. The Twelve Step program helps people deal with these emotions by teaching them how to find their spirituality.

I am hardly the first person to suggest that the Twelve Steps can benefit those with chronic illnesses. Many others whose lives have been transformed by a Twelve Step program have applied these principles to conditions ranging from cancer to AIDS.

However, what has been lacking in these interpretations is a plan for individual conditions. Until now.

This book is part of the Hazelden Pocket Health Guide series, a series of books that adapts the Twelve Steps for those with chronic illnesses—in this case, hypertension, also known as high blood pressure. The book combines specific medical guidelines with a plan to improve emotional and spiritual well-being. At its core is a program of hope, happiness, and healing.

Above all, this program provides those with chronic illnesses such as hypertension what they need: the indispensable tools and inspiration to live life one day at a time . . . and to *live it well*.

Spirituality:
The Strongest Medicine of All?

Can spirituality help me beat my disease? That's probably the question you're asking yourself. A better question might be, Can the spiritual program this book teaches help me manage my disease more effectively? The answer to that question is "yes."

The National Institutes of Health recognizes spirituality as an important component of alternative and complementary medicine. No wonder. A growing body of evidence suggests that spirituality actually helps people stay healthy and recover from illness.

In one of the most extensive laboratory studies ever done on the subject of spirituality and disease, researchers at Harvard's Mind/Body Medical Institute recently found that prayer and meditation—prerequisites for a sound spiritual life—cause a person's body to undergo healthful changes.[1] Metabolism, heart rate, and rate of breathing decrease, and brain waves slow down. These changes are the opposite of those induced by stress and are an effective therapy for certain

---

1. For a brochure describing the Mind/Body Medical Institute, call (617) 632-9525 or visit its Web site at www.mindbody.harvard.edu

diseases, especially those chronic in nature. Significantly, many doctors believe that because stress worsens a disease, a spiritual program that involves prayer and meditation is an effective component of treatment. If this is true, it is only logical to conclude that spirituality benefits those who have hypertension.

Although skeptics still question whether the chronically ill person who is spiritual is more likely to benefit medically than someone who is not spiritual, of this there is no doubt: spirituality helps chronically ill people cope with the emotional challenges of their condition.

But just what is spirituality, anyway? Spirituality is an inherent belief in the existence of a Higher Power, energy, or force—one that a person may or may not choose to call God—and a feeling of closeness to that entity. We experience that feeling of closeness, or connection, through the quality of our relationships with self, others, and our Higher Power. When we take the time and effort to communicate with our Higher Power through prayer and meditation and to treat others and ourselves with kindness, we strengthen connection—we feel spirituality at work.

That being is referred to variously within these pages as a Higher Power, a Power greater than ourselves, or as a Power Greater.

This book advocates use of the Twelve Steps, a

spiritual program founded in the 1930s to help alcoholics recover from the disease of alcoholism. The Twelve Steps can help you "turn over" care of your disease to a Higher Power that is greater and wiser than you, and that loves you. The program will help you maintain strength and hope as you live each day with your disease.

You'll learn in depth about the Twelve Steps later in this book. Right now what's important is that you know that managing your hypertension isn't just about arresting the medical aspects of the disease, although you will certainly learn most of what you need to know in these pages. No, recovery from hypertension is also about living well with that chronic illness every day.

The Twelve Steps will help you do this by allowing you to recognize what you do and don't have control over. In cooperation with your Higher Power, you have the wisdom to deal with your feelings about your disease and to change the behaviors that caused or exacerbated the condition, as well as to take certain steps to prevent it from getting worse, such as exercising, changing your diet, and taking your medication. The Twelve Steps will also show you how to grow spiritually through prayer, meditation, and support.

There may be no cure for hypertension, just as there is no cure for alcoholism and other chronic illnesses. However, if you practice the principles outlined in the

Twelve Steps, they will provide you with the resolve you need to control your hypertension—and with a way of life you may never have experienced had you not been stricken with a chronic illness.

Despite their popularity, Twelve Step programs are still widely misunderstood in some quarters. Such misunderstandings stand in the way of their acceptance by those who could really use them, including people with chronic illnesses such as hypertension. Perhaps the most common misunderstanding is that Twelve Step programs are "covers" for religion and, specifically, Christian groups.

A hasty reading of the Steps may reinforce this impression. However, reading more carefully you'll discover that the Steps do not endorse any religion. A person who lives by the Steps could be Jewish, Christian, Hindu, Muslim, Buddhist, agnostic.

If the Twelve Steps are not a religious program, then they certainly are a spiritual one. The Steps echo what writer Aldous Huxley called the "perennial philosophy"—a core set of ideas and practices shared by many religious traditions. The Steps have one major concern and that is human transformation.

You may already be intimately familiar with a Twelve Step program. If you have not experienced the Steps, you will discover that they offer a new approach to living. This approach is available to you if you acknowledge your jeopardy and your need to change your behaviors and to improve your state of being.

The spiritual component of this book draws extensively on principles developed by the founders of Alcoholics Anonymous. Like alcoholism, hypertension is a chronic disease. It is always with you, even when your blood pressure isn't elevated. And as with alcoholics, if you don't do what's necessary to address your condition, your disease will profoundly affect your life.

Alcoholics must abstain from alcohol and other drugs. As a person with hypertension—depending on the cause of your condition—you must be active, eat a nutritious diet, and take your medication regularly. The extraordinary success achieved by millions of participants in Twelve Step programs who now abstain from alcohol and other drugs can be emulated by those with hypertension who follow the Steps suggested in this book.

It is heartening to know that the Promises that inspire Alcoholics Anonymous members also offer strength and hope to people with hypertension who are willing to follow this simple program:

> If we are painstaking about this phase of our development, we will be amazed before we are half way through. We are going to know a new freedom and a new happiness. We will not regret the past

nor wish to shut the door on it. We will comprehend the word serenity and we will know peace. No matter how far down the scale we have gone, we will see how our experience can benefit others. That feeling of uselessness and self-pity will disappear. We will lose interest in selfish things and gain interest in our fellows. Self-seeking will slip away. Our whole attitude and outlook upon life will change. Fear of people and of economic insecurity will leave us. We will intuitively know how to handle situations which used to baffle us. We will suddenly realize that God is doing for us what we could not do for ourselves.[2]

The Twelve Step program of spirituality discussed in this book stresses acceptance. Only when you accept that you have hypertension and that it can cause serious health consequences will you be able to take the steps necessary to address the disease. Not only will denial prevent you from addressing the spiritual component of your chronic disease but also in a very real way it will delay you from taking the vital medical measures necessary to improve and extend your life. Thus, the first part of this book describes the chronic disease of hypertension, its symptoms, causes, and treatment.

2. *Alcoholics Anonymous*, 3d ed. (New York: AA World Services, Inc., 1976), 83–84. Reprinted with permission.

The Twelve Steps for Hypertension[3]

Step One—We admitted we were powerless over chronic illness—that our lives had become unmanageable.

Step Two—Came to believe that a Power greater than ourselves could restore us to sanity.

Step Three—Made a decision to turn our will and our lives over to the care of a Power greater than ourselves.

Step Four—Made a searching and fearless moral inventory of ourselves.

Step Five—Admitted to the God of our understanding, to ourselves, and to another human being the exact nature of our wrongs.

Step Six—Were entirely ready to have the God of our understanding remove all these defects of character.

Step Seven—Humbly asked our Higher Power to remove our shortcomings.

Step Eight—Made a list of all persons we had harmed, and became willing to make amends to them all.

Step Nine—Made direct amends to such people wherever possible, except when to do so would injure them or others.

3. Adapted from the Twelve Steps of Alcoholics Anonymous with the permission of AA World Services, Inc., New York, N.Y.

Step Ten—Continued to take personal inventory and when we were wrong promptly admitted it.

Step Eleven—Sought through prayer and meditation to improve our conscious contact with a Power greater than ourselves, praying only for knowledge of our Higher Power's will and the courage to carry that out.

Step Twelve—Having had a spiritual awakening as the result of these Steps, we tried to carry our message to others with our condition and to practice these principles in all our affairs.

The Twelve Steps of Alcoholics Anonymous[4]

Step One—We admitted we were powerless over alcohol—that our lives had become unmanageable.

Step Two—Came to believe that a Power greater than ourselves could restore us to sanity.

Step Three—Made a decision to turn our will and our lives over to the care of God *as we understood Him.*

Step Four—Made a searching and fearless moral inventory of ourselves.

---

4. The Twelve Steps of AA are taken from *Alcoholics Anonymous,* 3d ed., published by AA World Services, Inc., New York, N.Y., 59–60. Reprinted with the permission of AA World Services, Inc. (See editor's note on copyright page.)

Step Five—Admitted to God, to ourselves, and to another human being the exact nature of our wrongs.

Step Six—Were entirely ready to have God remove all these defects of character.

Step Seven—Humbly asked Him to remove our shortcomings.

Step Eight—Made a list of all persons we had harmed, and became willing to make amends to them all.

Step Nine—Made direct amends to such people wherever possible, except when to do so would injure them or others.

Step Ten—Continued to take personal inventory and when we were wrong promptly admitted it.

Step Eleven—Sought through prayer and meditation to improve our conscious contact with God *as we understood Him,* praying only for knowledge of His will for us and the power to carry that out.

Step Twelve—Having had a spiritual awakening as the result of these steps, we tried to carry this message to alcoholics, and to practice these principles in all our affairs.

CHAPTER ONE

Hypertension Essentials

Hypertension is a disease whose chief characteristic is high blood pressure. High blood pressure occurs when the blood being pumped from your heart pushes too hard against the walls of your veins. Throughout this book the terms "hypertension" and "high blood pressure" will be used interchangeably. Hypertension has reached epidemic proportions. An estimated fifty million Americans suffer from this condition, which in the vast majority of cases is irreversible. Hypertension greatly increases your chance of getting heart or kidney disease, or of having a stroke. This is deadly serious. Heart disease is the number-one killer in the United States, and stroke is the third most common cause of death.

Although the precise causes of most hypertension cases are unknown, factors that are thought to contribute to the most common form of hypertension include alcohol consumption, smoking, stress, and diet.

Hypertension is an incurable disease. However, when you take action to keep your blood pressure down, you minimize the danger of the disease. Living a full and healthy life with hypertension requires a willingness to maintain a healthy lifestyle that will keep your blood pressure at a healthy level.

Because people with hypertension experience no pain or other noticeable symptoms for many years, fewer than 25 percent of those with this condition are satisfactorily diagnosed and treated. Even those who have received attention for their condition often neglect to take their medication or to modify their lifestyle because they experience no obvious benefit from doing so.

Seemingly benign and yet so deadly, hypertension has been called the silent killer.

What Is Blood Pressure and What Happens When It Is High?

Blood is carried from the heart to all your body's tissues and organs in vessels called arteries. Blood pressure is the force of the blood pushing against the walls of those arteries. Each time the heart beats (about sixty to seventy times per minute at rest), it pumps blood into the arteries.

Blood pressure is measured in terms of systolic and diastolic pressure. Systolic is the blood pressure level when the heart is contracting to pump blood. Diastolic indicates the blood pressure level when the heart is at rest.

Different activities make your blood pressure go up or down. For example, running to catch the subway will elevate your blood pressure. On the other hand, when you're asleep, your blood pressure is relatively low. These changes in blood pressure are normal.

Some people have blood pressure that is high all or most of the time. Their blood pushes against the walls of their arteries with higher-than-normal force. If untreated this can lead to one or more of the following serious medical problems:

- Arteriosclerosis ("hardening of the arteries"): High blood pressure thickens and stiffens the walls of the arteries, making them less efficient in washing through substances such as fat and cholesterol. This accelerates the buildup of cholesterol and fats in the blood vessels (like rust in a pipe), which prevents enough blood from flowing through the body, and in time can lead to a heart attack or stroke.
- Heart attack: Blood carries oxygen to cells throughout the body. When the arteries that bring blood to the heart muscle become blocked, the heart does not get enough oxygen. Reduced

blood flow can cause chest pain (angina). Eventually, the flow may be stopped completely, causing a heart attack.

- Enlarged heart: High blood pressure causes the heart to work harder. Over time, the heart thickens and stretches. Eventually, the heart fails to pump blood normally, and fluids back up into the lungs.
- Kidney damage: The kidneys act as a filter to rid the body of wastes. Gradually, high blood pressure can narrow and thicken the blood vessels of the kidneys. The kidneys then filter less fluid, and waste builds up in the blood. The kidneys may fail altogether. When this happens, medical treatment (dialysis) or a kidney transplant may be needed.
- Stroke: High blood pressure can thicken the arteries to the brain, making them too narrow for normal blood flow. This can deprive the brain of enough blood and can also cause blood to clot in the narrowed arteries. If a blood clot blocks one of the narrowed arteries, a thrombiotic stroke may occur. A hemorrhagic stroke can occur when very high pressure causes a stiffened blood vessel in the brain to break.

Causes of Hypertension

The three types of hypertension are defined according to their causes.

Primary Hypertension

By far the most common form of hypertension is primary hypertension (sometimes called essential or idiopathic hypertension). Its precise cause is unknown, though a family history of hypertension is considered the most important risk factor for this condition. If both your parents have hypertension, it's likely you will develop the condition.

Other factors that contribute to the development of primary hypertension are

- poor diet (especially one high in salt, fat, and calories, and low in fruit, vegetables, and low-fat dairy products)
- obesity
- lack of exercise
- race (high blood pressure incidence is highest in people of African origin and lowest in people of East Asian origin)

Are You a Candidate for Hypertension?

Do you think you may have high blood pressure but have not spoken with a doctor about it?

Then consider the following questions related to your medical history:

- *Have you ever taken medication for high blood pressure but quit?*
- *Do you have a family history of hypertension or heart disease?*
- *Are you a woman who takes birth control medication?*
- *Are you of a race or an ethnic group that is at greater risk of developing hypertension (African Americans are at especially high risk of developing high blood pressure)?*

Consider also the following questions related to your lifestyle:

- *Do you drink alcoholic beverages regularly or excessively?*
- *Do you smoke?*
- *Do you get little or no regular physical exercise?*
- *Are you overweight for your height and build?*
- *Do you eat a lot of salty foods or add a lot of salt to your food?*
- *Is your diet high in cholesterol and/or saturated fats?*

If you answer yes to any of these questions, it is essential you consult a doctor. The information in this book can help prepare you for that visit.

Secondary Hypertension

If a person's hypertension is related to a specific medical problem, the condition is known as secondary hypertension. The most frequent cause of secondary hypertension is kidney (renal) disorder. Other conditions, such as tumors of the adrenal gland, chronic kidney disease, and hormone abnormalities, can cause hypertension too. Often, if the disease causing the hypertension is treated successfully, the hypertension goes away.

Certain medications can also cause high blood pressure. When medication is the source of high blood pressure, it also falls under the category of secondary hypertension. Medications that contain hormones, including birth control pills and steroids, raise blood pressure in some patients. Alcohol consumption is a significant cause of secondary hypertension.

Renovascular Hypertension

A rare form of hypertension is renovascular hypertension. This condition is caused by the narrowing of one or both of the renal arteries—the main arteries supplying blood to the kidneys.

White-Coat Hypertension

In addition to the three forms of hypertension described on pages 5 and 7, there is a fourth category of high blood pressure called white-coat hypertension. It isn't as serious as the other forms of hypertension because it is, in fact, a "false" form of the condition and is only short-lived.

What is white-coat hypertension? It refers to the phenomenon in which the stress of a visit to the doctor in itself causes the blood pressure to rise so much that a high blood pressure reading is recorded.

This phenomenon implies that significant numbers of people are being treated for a serious disease they do not have. It should be emphasized, however, that for every person being treated for a disease he or she doesn't have, there are several others who have the disease but aren't being treated. Hypertension is a disease that suffers from underdiagnosis, not false alarms.

People who measure their blood pressure at home using a sphygmomanometer (a blood pressure cuff) need to be aware that in a clinical setting their blood pressure readings may be significantly higher than they are when taken at home.

Who Is Likely to Develop High Blood Pressure?

Anyone can develop high blood pressure, but some people are more likely to get it than others. For example, high blood pressure is more common, develops earlier, and is more severe in people of African descent than in people of European descent.

In the early and middle adult years, men are more likely to have high blood pressure than women, but the reverse becomes true as men and women age. After age sixty-five, more women have high blood pressure than men. Whether you're a man or woman, the older you get, the more likely you are to develop high blood pressure; more than half of all Americans over age sixty-five are hypertensive.

Finally, hypertension is hereditary, which makes some families more prone to getting high blood pressure. If your parents or grandparents had high blood pressure, your risk may be increased.

Hypertension in Children

While mainly a disease of adults, high blood pressure can occur in children as well. Experts estimate 10 to 15 percent of school-age children have hypertension. Indeed, the condition is the most common reason student athletes fail sports pre-participation exams.

The American Heart Association recommends that children have their blood pressure checked annually.

Primary hypertension, the most common form of high blood pressure in both children and adults, usually has no clear cause. Common risk factors for children, however, are

• *obesity*
• *heredity*
• *race*

In rare cases, kidney or heart problems cause secondary hypertension in children. Physicians prefer not to use medication to treat primary hypertension in children. Instead, efforts are made to have children lower their high blood pressure by losing weight, decreasing salt intake, and exercising.

Symptoms of Hypertension

People with hypertension often write off the disease. They may say, "So what if I have high blood pressure?" Unfortunately, they eventually come to find out that hypertension causes havoc as the elevated blood pressure starts interfering with how their major organs work.

It's important to understand that it takes between ten and thirty years before this insidious disease causes serious symptoms. People with hypertension walk around for years without noticing any symptoms whatsoever. The only knowledge of their disease comes from a blood pressure reading. In part, this explains why a blood pressure check is always done when a person visits a clinic or hospital.

Symptoms do occur when blood pressure has been elevated for many years and has caused organ damage, so-called end-stage hypertension. End-stage hypertension symptoms include headaches, palpitations, dizziness, nosebleeds, shortness of breath, chest pain, or just plain fatigue.

Of course, several other conditions can cause these symptoms, so it is important for a doctor to determine which condition is the true cause.

Understanding Blood Pressure Readings

Your blood pressure is at its greatest when the heart contracts to pump out blood. This is called systolic pressure. Your blood pressure falls when the heart is at rest between beats. This is called diastolic pressure.

Blood pressure readings consist of these two numbers—the systolic and diastolic pressures—one on top of the other, with the top number always being the systolic pressure. An example of a blood pressure reading is 120/80 mm Hg (millimeters of mercury), which would be expressed verbally as "120 over 80."

High blood pressure is classified by stages and is more serious as the numbers get higher. Table 1.1 contains the most up-to-date system doctors use to classify people's blood pressure.[1]

---

1. The numbers are based on an average of two readings done at separate times *after* the initial screening.

Condition	Systolic (top number)	Diastolic (bottom number)	What to Do
Normal	Less than 130	Less than 85	Have your doctor recheck in two years.
High-normal	130–139	85–89	Have your doctor recheck in one year.
Hypertension: Stage 1	140–159	90–99	Have your doctor confirm diagnosis within two months.
Hypertension: Stage 2	160–179	100–109	Start treatment within one month.
Hypertension: Stage 3	180–209	110–119	Start treatment within one week.
Hypertension: Stage 4	210 or higher	120 or higher	Start treatment immediately!

Table 1.1 Classification of High Blood Pressure Readings

Diagnosing Hypertension

Because of the potential for false readings caused by white-coat hypertension, the cornerstone of diagnosing hypertension is taking a number of blood pressure readings over the course of a few weeks to make sure that a sustained elevation of pressure really exists. There are several ways of doing this, including repeated visits to the doctor's office, using a blood pressure cuff at home, or, sometimes, using a device that will continuously measure pressure over twenty-four hours.

You have true hypertension only if your blood pressure is consistently high when you are resting comfortably and haven't done anything to raise your blood pressure. You should not smoke for one hour before having your blood pressure tested or consume alcohol for twelve hours before a reading.

Having your blood pressure checked is quick, easy, and painless. A blood pressure cuff is wrapped around your upper arm and inflated to stop the blood flow in your artery for a few seconds. Then a valve is opened and the air is released from the cuff. This removes the pressure and a stethoscope records the blood rushing back through the artery. The first sound heard and registered on the gauge, or mercury column, is the systolic pressure, followed by the diastolic pressure.

If your blood pressure reading on your initial exam is high, your doctor will probably schedule further tests to confirm the reading. In the meantime, he or she may give you a physical exam to determine whether a specific cause for your probable hypertension can be found. Your doctor should check to see whether hypertension has damaged blood vessels in your brain, heart, kidneys, or other organs. Your doctor will also ask about risk factors, including a family history of hypertension, stroke, and heart disease; alcohol consumption; smoking; cholesterol levels; and diabetes.

How to Prepare for a Physical Exam

Before you see your doctor about hypertension, it is a good idea to make a list of any symptoms, questions, or concerns that you may have. Also, be prepared to discuss your family medical history.

What exactly happens during a physical examination for hypertension? A physical examination for hypertension may include the following:

- *Two or more blood pressure determinations in three positions: seated, standing, and lying down*
- *Thorough eye examination to check for signs of retinal disease related to hypertension, a condition that can cause degenerative changes in the eye*
- *Examination of the neck with a stethoscope to listen for unusual sounds in the arteries, swollen neck veins, and enlarged thyroid*
- *Examination of the heart to check for evidence*

of an enlarged heart, abnormal heart sounds (murmurs), irregular heartbeats, and other signs that indicate possible heart disease
- *Examination of the chest to listen for abnormal lung sounds*
- *Examination of the abdomen*
- *Examination of the arms and legs for weak or absent pulses and swelling*
- *Neurological examination*

What laboratory tests are performed? Some include the following:

- *Complete blood count (CBC)*
- *Serum chemistry, including potassium, creatinine, and magnesium*
- *Urinalysis*
- *Fasting blood sugar*
- *Fasting lipoprotein profile (low-density lipoprotein [LDL], high-density lipoprotein [HDL], cholesterol, and triglycerides)*
- *Electrocardiography (ECG or EKG)*
- *Chest radiography*

Depending on the results of these tests and an assessment of your condition, your doctor may order more specific tests.

Hypertension: Incurable but Controllable

Primary hypertension cannot be cured. It is a disease you have for life. Furthermore, it's a disease that will kill you unless you take the measures necessary to control it. Fortunately, when your blood pressure is kept down, the danger of your hypertension is minimized. The key is your willingness to do what's necessary to keep your blood pressure at a healthy level.

Once an accurate diagnosis is made, the most important goal is to establish a time period within which to bring your condition under control permanently. These are the components of a successful program to address the physical and psychological symptoms of your hypertension:

- Improve diet.
- Lose weight.
- Increase daily activity; begin an exercise program.
- Abstain from alcohol; limit alcohol consumption.
- Stop smoking.
- Follow appropriate drug therapy.
- Avoid medications that raise blood pressure such as birth control pills and nonsteroidal anti-inflammatories (Motrin, Aleve, etc.).
- Treat addictions to substances such as alcohol, cocaine, and methamphetamine.
- Commit to a spiritual program.

Hypertension: The Mind-Body Connection

Strong evidence suggests that spirituality is a key to extending survival rates for chronic illness. People with hypertension have responded especially well to spiritual programs. A by-product of these programs is to bring participants to a relaxed and peaceful state, a condition from which people with hypertension can certainly benefit. In addition to the physical benefits, practicing the principles of a spiritual program is known to enhance a person's ability to cope emotionally with chronic conditions such as hypertension.

Such coping skills are greatly needed. People diagnosed with hypertension may have difficulty accepting either that they have the disease or that it has serious consequences. As a result, they don't take the necessary measures to control it. Acceptance is an integral component of an effective spiritual program for chronic illness. If and when a person does accept the diagnosis of hypertension, emotions such as anger, frustration, anxiety, and depression are apt to surface. A spiritual program for chronic illness will help alleviate such feelings.

The medical profession is at last coming to recognize the need for a spiritual component in the management of chronic illnesses such as hypertension. No less an institution than Harvard Medical School is dedicated to studying this phenomenon. The doctors at the

Mind/Body Medical Institute at Harvard have discovered in laboratory studies that prayer and meditation actually lower blood pressure. Although not all doctors are as open-minded as the physicians at the Mind/Body Institute, the health care profession is beginning to acknowledge the great gift available to those people with chronic illness who commit to exploring their spirituality.

Effects of High Blood Pressure

High blood pressure is known as the "silent killer." It does not have recognizable symptoms but, left untreated, can cause severe damage to major organs, including the brain and the heart.

- In the brain, blood vessels can become blocked or can burst, causing a stroke.
- Vision worsens due to narrowed blood vessels in the eyes.
- Blood vessels become less pliable and may narrow due to a buildup of fatty deposits.
- Increased pressure in blood vessels causes the heart to strain and grow larger, increasing risk of angina (chest pain caused by inadequate blood flow through the blood vessels of the heart), heart attack, or heart failure.
- Kidneys can become damaged from hardening and narrowing of blood vessels.

To avoid the serious consequences associated with hypertension, it's extremely important to adhere to doctor recommendations concerning lifestyle changes and medication, regardless of how well you may feel.

CHAPTER TWO

A Spiritual Program
to Help Manage Hypertension

Treatment to control your hypertension is available. You just need to find out what to do and do it. So what's the problem?

It is a challenge to make the changes in your life that are necessary to manage hypertension. But if you have hypertension, change holds the promise of rewards beyond that of just lowering your blood pressure. Change provides you with the opportunity to learn to live a life that is more happy, joyous, and free—a life that may be better than you've ever known.

The question is, How do you go about this?

To achieve the resolve you need to successfully address your disease, you need a spiritual plan as well as a medical one. The Twelve Step program referred to throughout the book is such a spiritual program. It has worked with astonishing success for millions of people with the chronic illnesses of addiction, including alcoholics and drug addicts, gamblers, and overeaters. Its principles have provided great succor for people with other chronic illnesses as well.

The Twelve Step program is at its core spiritual. It is strictly nondenominational, however, and accommodates people of all faiths. The program also welcomes those who do not have religious faith. Nevertheless, success in this program requires a profound change in thinking from self-centeredness to acceptance of a Higher Power beyond oneself.

How you see your Higher Power is a matter of personal choice. It does not have to be God in a traditional sense. If you asked individuals whose lives have been positively transformed by the Twelve Steps to identify their Higher Power, you would get a variety of answers. Many people would undoubtedly tell you that the most meaningful aspect of believing in a Higher Power was to be able to step outside themselves and realize they were not the center of everything.

Twelve Step How-To

Thanks to the foresight of those who created the Twelve Step program, there is flexibility in this guide to better living with chronic illness. This set of principles makes no draconian demands on you but rather offers suggestions for behavioral changes that will result in an improved life with less emotional pain and greater spirituality.

There is no rule about how the Steps should be done. This is a matter of personal preference. Many people with chronic illnesses have experienced great improvement in their spiritual well-being by choosing to do the Steps selectively. However, the Twelve Steps build on each other. If you take the time to get a firm foothold on one Step before you go on to the next, you journey from acceptance to serenity one Step at a time.

Many people ask, Is there a time frame for doing the Steps? As long as it takes is probably the best advice. But it is important to feel you are making progress. As far as possible, you need not feel stalled on one Step or take lengthy breaks between Steps.

And keep in mind that doing the Steps isn't a one-time thing. You continue to practice the principles of the Steps in your daily life, and there is nothing to stop you from starting again on Step One and working all the way to Step Twelve whenever you wish. For many people, "working the Steps" provides tremendous serenity and satisfaction, not to mention a simple plan for living well.

A careful reading of this chapter will reveal that the underlying concepts of the Twelve Steps are not unique. Those who developed the Twelve Steps simply reflected on how they got sober. But their experience is supported by the collective sagacity of philosophers, cultures, and religious leaders throughout the ages. You will soon see that the message in the Steps is ageless;

the philosophy is timeless; and the strength and hope offered to those with chronic illnesses such as hypertension are everlasting.

Much has been written about the Twelve Steps. The following pages will introduce you to each Step. If this is your first encounter with the Steps, you may find it helpful to gather more information. If you've been exposed to the Steps or currently work the program for an addiction, this chapter can serve as a review.

Step One: The Foundation of Recovery

We admitted we were powerless over chronic illness— that our lives had become unmanageable.

We've probably all heard it said that the first step is the hardest to take. This is certainly true with the Twelve Steps. In taking Step One, we must admit that we are powerless over hypertension and that a most important part of our lives—our health—is out of control. Who wants to do such a thing?

Step One gets us to face reality. We cannot alter the fact that we have hypertension. We suffer from a disease that is incurable. We can take measures to minimize the harmful effects of our hypertension, but the disease is always part of who we are. We are powerless to change that fact.

We also need to realize that something in our lives has become unmanageable. That something—whether a stressful situation, poor meal planning, lack of exercise, or neglecting our health—may be exacerbating our high blood pressure. If we're not taking care of ourselves—whether by dealing with our problems or by taking care of our bodies—we're not seeing our health as a priority. That alone can be the stepping-stone for all sorts of unmanageability in our lives. If we don't feel good ourselves, we have trouble caring for others and doing our jobs.

The First Step takes courage. We have to admit things about ourselves that we would prefer not to, and we have to see that our choices have produced consequences. Admitting that we have to take measures to deal with our chronic illness is the best way to go forward. Like thousands who have gone before us, we can summon the courage we need to take this Step, the first in our spiritual journey toward achieving the serenity we need to manage our disease in its entirety.

Step Two: A Promise of Hope

Came to believe that a Power greater than ourselves could restore us to sanity.

Spirituality is an integral part of any Twelve Step program for chronic illness. Why? Because finding the serenity and strength we need to manage this disease requires turning to a power beyond ourselves.

Many of us already believe in a Higher Power we

call God. If we don't believe in a Power greater than ourselves, it's important we at least stay open-minded about the concept. Even the slightest amount of faith that a Higher Power can and will help us is better than no faith at all. If this proves difficult, we "act as if" we believe so we're open to experiencing its power.

Indeed, Step Two does not mean we must come to believe in God as presented in a formal religious context. If we think this is the case, we might dismiss the Twelve Step program because we think it won't work for us. Or, if we're religious, we may view the Steps as some sort of cult. We need to keep an open mind. Like all the Steps, Step Two is a suggestion from others who say, "This is the way it worked for us." These people have found that the Second Step gave them hope—and there is hope for us if we come to believe that the source of power we need lies outside ourselves.

If we were to ask all the people with hypertension who have been restored to sanity how they identify their Higher Power, we would probably hear answers as varied as humankind's ideas on faith. Some might say God as they understand Him from the faith of their upbringing (the Christian God, for example); some may be more comfortable envisioning a female version of God; others might say God working through the Twelve Step program; and others might say their Power Greater was the Twelve Steps themselves, along with support group attendance and fellowship. A Higher Power is meaningful and personal, an entity with whom we find a powerful connection.

On Insanity

"Restore me to sanity? But I'm not insane!" That might be your response to the second part of Step Two. Insanity here refers to our tendency to steadfastly refuse to acknowledge our hypertension—even after we've been told that unless we do something, we'll suffer deadly consequences. The *American Heritage Dictionary* defines "insane" as being foolish or absurd. Most people would agree that not taking the clear-cut measures necessary to control a life-threatening disease meets the definition of foolish or absurd.

Step Three: Turning It Over

Made a decision to turn our will and our lives over to the care of a Power greater than ourselves.

Of all the Steps, the Third Step can be the most effective in helping us transcend the emotional pain of chronic illness. Time and time again Step Three has provided what people have needed to get through difficult moments. It has helped them approach the management of their disease with remarkable resolve.

In Step One we admit we are powerless over the fact that we have hypertension, and we acknowledge that our disease has made our lives unmanageable. In Step Two we come to believe that a Higher Power can help us get through our emotional pain. Step Three is making the decision to let our Higher Power relieve us from the emotional pain and unmanageability of our disease and show us what we can do ourselves.

Turning our will over to a Power greater than ourselves doesn't absolve us from doing whatever is necessary to care for ourselves. Our Higher Power loves us whatever we do and helps us by showing us how to help ourselves. Our Higher Power speaks through others and through us. We learn to listen to our feelings and to act on them.

No longer will we try to force impossible solutions or beliefs that aren't in our best interest. We won't expend time and energy "willing" our disease to go away. We let our Higher Power determine the best way for us to handle our disease and all the emotions that go along with it.

It is the responsibility of each and every one of us with hypertension to cooperate with our Higher Power. We need to do all we can to improve ourselves physically, mentally, spiritually, and emotionally.

Turning our will and our lives over to the care of a Higher Power doesn't "cure" our hypertension. But it does help us handle the challenge of managing our disease. It gives us the ability to consider a plan or purpose higher than our own.

Achieving the balance between letting our Higher Power care for us and taking personal responsibility can be hard. We discover how to achieve this balance by communicating with our Higher Power through prayer and meditation. In this way the answers are often revealed.

Once we have begun the process of "turning it over," we begin to find the resolve to manage our hypertension. We can halt, go inside ourselves, and in the tranquillity simply say the Serenity Prayer: "God, grant me the serenity to accept the things I cannot change, the courage to change the things I can, and the wisdom to know the difference. Thy will, not mine, be done."

Spirituality

Just what is spirituality, anyway? One thing it isn't is religion. Although many truly religious people are spiritual, and many spiritual people consider themselves to be religious, the two concepts are not one and the same. We don't have to be religious to be spiritual. Religion is a codification of society's relationship with God into rituals and institutions. Spirituality is our inherent relationship with ourselves, others, and a Higher Power.

Step Four: Knowing Yourself

Made a searching and fearless moral inventory of ourselves.

The importance of doing an inventory is to know ourselves better. By being searching and fearless about our liabilities, we gain insight into how we may have developed the disease hypertension and why we react the way we do. Writing down an inventory helps us to understand what we need to do to correct the behaviors that have brought us to this point, and which ways of living will best help us manage our disease.

In doing this Step, we must be moral but not moralistic. Our behavior has been good and bad—that is the reality. We must examine it. Make it ours. For example, many of us didn't exercise for many years, or perhaps we ate, smoked, and drank to excess. Neglecting our health was selfish and self-centered. Number one, we ignored the impact our poor health would have on our families. Think about it. And what about pride? We may have refused to acknowledge that our high blood pressure readings meant we were "really" sick— after all, we didn't have any symptoms. We also need to examine our behavior since being diagnosed with hypertension. Have we indulged in excessive self-pity and ignored our doctors' recommendations? Have we taken our frustrations and displeasure out on our families and friends? Do we continue to overeat, smoke, or drink, or not exercise?

In doing our inventories, we shouldn't restrict ourselves to aspects of our behavior having only to do with our hypertension. It is important for us that we recognize flaws that may have nothing to do with whether we developed high blood pressure.

We mustn't punish ourselves for these behaviors. The goal is to know ourselves and to accept ourselves. Only when we see ourselves in a way that is enlightening, and not judgmental, can we strive to do better.

There are several ways to go about Step Four. The most common way is to use a straightforward, double-column list of specific positive and negative behaviors. Keep in mind that Step Four is not a test. We cannot fail it.

Taking the Fourth Step is a profound yet simple start to an ongoing way of daily living. It is the beginning of a path to self-awareness, a way to go today and each day hereafter. The inventory becomes a way of life based on the courage and willingness to be completely honest to oneself about oneself.

This self-assessment may be the most difficult feat of our lives. If we need encouragement, support, or help, we can ask for it from someone we trust, such as a chaplain or counselor—someone who will be nonjudgmental.

When we have completed our Fourth Step inventories, we will possess more self-awareness and self-acceptance. We're now ready for the Fifth Step. We're now ready to make some changes in our lives and in the ways we manage our disease.

Step Five: Telling My Story

Admitted to the God of our understanding, to ourselves, and to another human being the exact nature of our wrongs.

In the Fifth Step, we openly, honestly, and willingly share who we are. This is a time for introspection as well as for laying ourselves bare. It allows us to let our Higher Power and another person see us for who we really are—flawed but lovable people capable of taking the measures necessary to manage hypertension.

Step Five gives us the chance to rid ourselves of the hidden side of ourselves, the side that sometimes causes us to feel shame.

We need to prepare for this Step. True self-awareness and honesty do not come easily to most people. We are used to avoiding our character defects. To stand and actually face ourselves as we truly are is a difficult and spiritually demanding proposition.

The key to a good Step Five is to have done a thorough, balanced, and honest Fourth Step. In particular, the rigorous self-honesty called for in Step Four helps us to gain the humility we need to do an effective Step Five.

To Admit to a Higher Power

With the help of a Higher Power, we can find the inner courage and strength we need to take the Fifth Step. Caring, loving, and forgiving, our Higher Power will help us realize that we are not the only ones who fall short.

To Admit to Ourselves

To admit to ourselves where we went wrong is a sign that we are practicing true self-honesty. But it isn't easy. Who wants to confess to character flaws that may have caused a chronic illness? We go through our lives ignoring the ways we inflicted damage on our own bodies. Really, though, we do not forget. The knowledge gnaws inside us.

Taking the Fifth Step without being totally self-honest is self-defeating. It merely perpetuates our dislike of ourselves.

To do this Step well it is important to love and to respect ourselves. Step Five allows us to reflect on whether we are coping with our disease in a loving and nonjudgmental way. It gives us the chance to accept ourselves as flawed human beings. It lets us understand that we need forgiveness and another chance at life. When we forgive ourselves, we become free from the grip of guilt and shame.

To admit first to ourselves before admitting to another person shows we are willing to be really honest. We prove we are not afraid to face our real selves squarely. True honesty begins with this kind of self-honesty. Knowing ourselves and our strengths and weaknesses can profoundly help us overcome any perceived obstacles to managing our hypertension.

To Admit to Another Person

We share the Fifth Step with another person. Why? Because sharing with another person the exact nature of our wrongs keeps us honest. By doing this Step, we allow another person to see us as complete, but flawed, human beings. Most of us will find this to be the hardest part of the Fifth Step. We may experience an overwhelming fear of embarrassment. But there is a great amount of relief in doing this. We no longer have to put energy into making others believe we're perfect.

Step Five is the opportunity to cast out those behaviors and traits that cause us emotional pain. It is not enough to acknowledge the nature of our wrongs to ourselves and through prayer to a Higher Power. It is only by speaking out, admitting out loud our mistakes, failures, and anxieties to another person that the feelings and deeds lose their power over us. For those of us with a chronic illness such as hypertension, the Fifth Step is one major step away from a sense of isolation and loneliness; it is a step toward wholeness, happiness, and a real sense of gratitude.

Which "Human Being"?

During Step Five, most people wonder, "With whom should I share my secrets?" The fact is that almost anyone will do: a clergy person, a doctor, a psychologist, a family member who won't be adversely affected by our total honesty, a counselor, a friend, or even a stranger. The best candidates have the following qualities:

- *discretion*
- *maturity and wisdom*
- *willingness to share their own experiences*
- *familiarity with the challenges of a chronic illness*

Often such people are not readily available to us. One of our responsibilities in doing the Fifth Step is to look around carefully for someone who meets these criteria.

Whomever we decide to share our Fifth Step with, we must remember our intention is not to please that person but to heal ourselves. It is our inner selves that we are trying to satisfy. We should also not be afraid of shocking listeners with our revelations.

Steps Four and Five Are Ongoing

The "housecleaning" process we do in Steps Four and Five is not meant to be a onetime event. As we will learn in Step Ten, regular personal inventories are measures we can take to help us transcend the emotional pain of our chronic disease and to better manage our condition. If and when we decide to do these Steps again, we do not need to go back over our whole lives unless we continue to carry anger or other unresolved feelings or realize we overlooked a behavior we would like to change. Otherwise, we pick up where we left off when we last took inventory. What is past is past. Whenever we take the Fourth and Fifth Steps again, it can become an opportunity for increasing our self-knowledge and self-acceptance, and for learning to forgive and seek forgiveness as a way of daily living.

Step Six: Ready, Willing, and Able

Were entirely ready to have the God of our understanding remove all these defects of character.

In Step One we admitted we were powerless over our

disease. In Step Two we came to believe that our Higher Power could help us. In Step Three we made the decision to let that Power care for our lives. Steps Four and Five uncovered our defects of character.

If we have done these first five Steps honestly and thoroughly, we will be ready to let go of our character defects. The readiness to have them removed is the key to the Sixth Step. By being willing to let go of these character defects, we increase our chances of coping with our chronic illness.

In taking Step Six, we need to revisit that concept of powerlessness. Instead of telling our Higher Power what we want to be—"Make me more motivated" or, "Make me more open-minded"—we state our condition as it is. We state how things are with us: "My Higher Power, I am lazy" or, "My Higher Power, I am intolerant of others." Only with this humility will we be ready and willing to have such defects removed.

Even with all the preparation we do for the Sixth Step, we may still have reservations. Even when we know we no longer have any use for our defects of character, we find that we've grown accustomed to them over the years. In our minds, our pride and selfishness served us well. We might ask ourselves, "Can I let go of some of my most monumental defects?"

That is why we go to the Seventh Step. It's there that we see our Higher Power doing for us what we really could not do for ourselves. For many, the removal of our shortcomings is the miracle that turns doubters into believers. Step Six is really the "get ready, get set" that builds toward the "go" of Step Seven—the action of asking our Higher Power to remove our shortcomings.

Step Seven: Being Changed

Humbly asked our Higher Power to remove our shortcomings.

The first word in Step Seven is "humbly." Because Step Seven so expressly concerns itself with humility, we need to stop to consider its importance.

Humility is the practice of being humble. It is the recognition of our self-worth and seeing that same God-given worth in other people, even when they are so totally unlike us that we don't understand them or get along with them. Humility is the awareness that we are not all-powerful controllers of every aspect of our lives and that we do need the help and guidance of a Higher Power.

"Humbly" asking our Higher Power is quite different from the way we may be used to praying—either begging or bargaining. In those cases we prayed to our Higher Power out of desperation. From now on we pray with humility; we humbly ask our Higher Power to remove our shortcomings.

Most people find it easier to ask that their short-comings be removed gradually or one at a time. Having lived with these shortcomings for so long, we may find it difficult to shed them all at once. We need to be patient with ourselves and with our Higher Power during this process. This may take time, a lot of work on our part, more of the being "entirely ready" of Step Six. We don't expect to become perfect people, but we aim to improve. The goal is progress, not perfection.

We can work this Step alone with our Higher Power, with members of a religious group, or in support groups (for alcoholism, nicotine addiction, or heart disease, for instance)—wherever we can trust and be trusted.

And although personal prayer is our own connection with our Higher Power, when two or three are gathered together, we feel a special bond not only with our Higher Power but also with others who share our condition. We feel this closeness as we say the Serenity Prayer together in our groups.

Our own shortcomings can, with our Higher Power's help, be changed.

Step Eight: Preparing for Change

Made a list of all persons we had harmed, and became willing to make amends to them all.

Step Eight adds even more strength to our program. If we have harmed others, it is important we get the guilt off our consciences and make a heartfelt attempt to reconcile with them. If we have hurt a friend and the friendship has suffered, the benefit is that we might repair that friendship. By making a list, we become clear as to exactly whom we owe amends to.

Over the years our personal habits such as drinking, smoking, and overeating may have caused discomfort to others—to family, friends, and co-workers. We may have been rude to them when they asked us to stop a particular behavior. Chances are that at the very least we ignored or rebuffed many people's feelings on the subject. Our smoking may have interfered with the family's social relations. Friends may not have wanted to come to our homes. Being lazy and unfit may have made some dream excursions or adventures out of the question.

We might want to consider what our behavior was like after we found out we had hypertension. It may have been unacceptable. We may have been disrespectful at times to the health professionals who were trying to help us with our recovery—doctors, nutritionists, exercise therapists. Our list needs to include all persons we've harmed, regardless of how much and under what circumstances.

We may want to put ourselves at the top of our

amends list. We are the ones whose health may be suffering as a result of our actions.

Understandably, the prospect of acknowledging our responsibility for hurting others can be daunting. As with the other Steps, Step Eight becomes less frightening once we settle down to do it.

We can take some time to write the names of a few people who make us feel uncomfortable. We don't need to write why, or anything else. The simple act of writing down names changes our perspective. Instead of thinking about the harm others have done to us, we take responsibility for the pain we caused in those relationships. It is a profound experience that represents a coming of age.

If you made a list, congratulations. You are halfway through this important Step.

Many of us avoid the Eighth Step because we are already thinking ahead to Step Nine or because we feel too guilty or fearful to face a long list of names. It is important to remember that just because we've written a list does not mean we need to make amends immediately.

The second part of this Step involves willingness. Being willing to make amends means discarding all resentments and accepting responsibility for the harm we have done to others.

In so doing we become completely ready to do

whatever we can to make amends for these harms, thereby unburdening ourselves of guilty feelings that interfere with our emotional well-being as we contend with our hypertension.

Continuing to Make Amends

The Twelve Step program is not a program of perfection. Instead, it stresses progress. Even when we practice the principles of this program in all our affairs, it is inevitable we will have "run-ins" with other people in our lives (though far fewer than before, it is hoped). For that reason a new and revised Step Eight list is an option for any of us at any time.

Step Nine: Facing the Past

Made direct amends to such people wherever possible, except when to do so would injure them or others.

We begin making amends to our loved ones by showing them we are caring for ourselves. In addition to starting an exercise program, we follow advice on nutrition, address nicotine and alcohol use, and, where necessary, learn to take our medications properly. No longer do our families and friends have to fear we are, through inaction, killing ourselves. We make many of our amends by taking appropriate measures to contain our disease.

These, though, are "indirect" amends, and the operative word in Step Nine is "direct." Making amends directly helps us gain humility, honesty, and courage. That means we need to go directly to the people we have harmed and admit our wrongs. Being direct isn't just about righting wrongs. It also inspires us to summon honesty and courage to our service and gives us the freedom to look others in the eye and to experience the self-respect we deserve.

An amend need not consist of a lengthy explanation. All that's needed is a heartfelt apology. The person to whom we are making the amend may feel some uneasiness too. For this reason, simplicity and directness usually work best when making the amend.

Ideally we apologize face-to-face. The very directness of this approach is beneficial. Sometimes this is impractical, however, and we may choose to write a letter, make a phone call, or even, in this electronic age, send an e-mail.

In the vast majority of cases, amends are well received. Even in those rare instances when they are not, this is not a reason to avoid the effort the next time. Almost always, relationships improve markedly when amends are made.

Steps Eight and Nine also allow us to make amends to ourselves. The reward for taking these Steps is a gradual but increasing sense of self-acceptance and self-respect, of being in harmony with our own personal world. Such feelings are indispensable in our quest to cope better with the challenges of our chronic illness.

Step Ten: Maintaining Our New Lives

Continued to take personal inventory and when we were wrong promptly admitted it.

Managing our chronic illness presents us with a tremendous challenge. Yet by following the Steps of this program, we have been able to achieve a strong measure of our relationships with ourselves, others, and a Higher Power. To help maintain our serenity, we must try to stay comfortable with ourselves and others. We do this by continuing to take a personal inventory.

We are only human. The path we are taking offers progress, not perfection, so it is inevitable—even with a Higher Power in our lives—that we will do things that we know are wrong or misguided. These acts can be monumental or trivial. Maybe if we have let our condition deteriorate to the point where distressing symptoms have begun, we entertained thoughts of suicide. Or the expense of a medication caused us to snap angrily at a pharmacist. When defects such as self-pity and anger rear up, we can go back and do a Seventh Step on them, asking our Higher Power to remove these shortcomings.

It helps to get feedback from people close to us—family members, friends, fellow participants of support groups. We need to ask these people to point out our character defects to us if they become apparent.

The second part of this Step emphasizes that if we want to maintain our serenity, we must admit our wrongs "promptly." It is important not to let anything build up inside us that will interfere with our program to cope with our chronic illness. Once we get used to it, admitting we're wrong can be a liberating sensation that enables us to move on in our lives without harboring resentments or other unhealthy thoughts.

Step Eleven: Partnership with a Higher Power

Sought through prayer and meditation to improve our conscious contact with a Power greater than ourselves, praying only for knowledge of our Higher Power's will and the courage to carry that out.

When coping with a chronic illness such as hypertension, we need all the help we can get. The help of a Power greater than ourselves is available to us through prayer (talking to our Higher Power) and meditation (listening to our Higher Power). By praying and meditating in our daily lives, we keep a channel open to our Higher Power. We can rely on that Power's strength to help us at any time as we deal with the challenges of our disease.

Step Eleven calls for us to follow our Higher Power's will as it is revealed to us through prayer and meditation. Once we believe we are trying to do our Higher Power's will, we can ask for the strength to carry that out. When we do not feel like exercising or eating properly, we can ask for encouragement. When we have a compulsion to drink or smoke, we can ask our Higher Power to take it away. Our Higher Power is always with us and willing to come to our aid.

It's important for us to remember that although we have turned over care of our disease to a Higher Power, we need to cooperate with that Power. By listening to others who share our condition, learning about our disease, and adhering to our doctors' advice, we are doing what is necessary to care for our hypertension and ourselves. We are acting as our Higher Power wishes us to act. And in so doing we are better able to receive the strength that Power wants to provide.

The Importance of Prayer and Meditation

Medical science has demonstrated that prayer and meditation have a beneficial effect on our health (see page xv). These practices improve our health by helping us develop a closer relationship with our Higher Power, an improved "spirit-consciousness."

Prayer is talking to our Higher Power.

Meditation is listening to our Higher Power. Prayer and meditation don't come easily to everyone. As with most things, the more we do it, the better we get. Those who have cultivated a close relationship with their Higher Power can suggest ways that we, too, can pray and meditate. We need to seek out such people and consult them or read books on how to meditate.

Perhaps the most oft-heard recommendation is to have a quiet time each morning during which we ask our Higher Power for the strength to manage our hypertension that day and a similar interlude each night when we thank our Higher Power for helping us to live another day with our chronic illness.

Many people meditate for at least thirty minutes a day—a duration we may need to work up to. Meditation involves quieting the mind. We can begin meditating by getting in a comfortable position, closing our eyes, and focusing on a word such as "peace." At first, many thoughts of what we "should" be doing enter our minds, but we learn to release them. When our minds are quiet, we are able to get in touch with our inner selves and to listen to our Higher Power. Afterward, sometimes miraculously, answers to our problems will just come to us.

The strength we need to cope with our

chronic illness comes from communicating with our Higher Power in prayer and meditation. We must actively seek out spirit-communication with our Higher Power. This is a matter directly between us and that Power. From direct communication comes life, joy, peace, and spiritual healing.

Step Twelve: Carrying the Message

Having had a spiritual awakening as the result of these Steps, we tried to carry our message to others with our condition and to practice these principles in all our affairs.

By the time we reach Step Twelve, we've changed. The compulsion to deny our disease and to engage in behaviors that caused it or made it worse has been lifted—not by our own power, but by a Power greater than ourselves. This in itself is a spiritual awakening that will help us as we contend with our disease.

If we've worked the Steps, we have the gift of being able to manage our chronic illness. If we haven't worked the program, we now know we have the tools.

Truly one of the best ways to keep this gift is to give it away. We have experience, strength, and hope that we can share with others. We let ourselves be used as a channel for a Higher Power to work through. We can now partake in the joy of helping others to live healthier, happier, and longer lives.

One way we might "give it away" is to make ourselves available as volunteers to those who organize heart disease prevention campaigns. Or we might provide comfort and company to people with heart disease living in convalescent homes. If we attend Alcoholics Anonymous or Nicotine Anonymous meetings, we can help make the coffee, set up beforehand, and clean up afterward.

If we belong to a heart disease support group and a member of our support group seems to be dwelling on the negative aspects of his or her life, we might take it upon ourselves to spend some time with this person and try to lend a sympathetic ear and an encouraging word.

Whether or not we find an organized support group, we need to seek out and make friends with two or more people with hypertension. We need to make it a point to have breakfast or lunch with them often, phone them regularly, and talk. We should praise their efforts and celebrate their successes (no matter how small) and let them do the same for us.

If we practice the principles of this Twelve Step program in all our affairs, we will likely realize our full physical potential with this disease and an abundance of spirit. We live as our Higher Power intends us to—happy, joyous, and free.

On Spiritual Awakenings

For those unfamiliar with Twelve Step programs, the term "spiritual awakening" can be the subject of confusion. Many people assume that a spiritual awakening is by definition a cataclysmic occurrence—an opening of the heavens accompanied by a chorus of hallelujahs. In the absence of such an event, some of us might assume the program isn't working for us. But instant and dramatic conversions to spirit-consciousness are not what the Twelve Steps are predicated on. Although such transformations take place, they are by no means the rule. Most spiritual awakenings are simple, very simple, and yet the feeling we experience is profound. We feel enlightened and in awe.

A spiritual awakening could be as simple as a thought we have while walking through the woods or watching a child. It could be suddenly seeing ourselves or others in a totally different light. It could be running into someone who gives us the answer to the question we've been asking ourselves.

A person may have one big spiritual awakening, but most people have many smaller-scale awakenings. As the Twelve Steps become our guide to living well with hypertension and as we develop a relationship with a Power greater than ourselves who loves us and cares for us, we come to an understanding of what is truly meant by the words "spiritual awakening."

Step by Step

We're now aware of the Twelve Steps and what they mean. They aren't always easy to accept or understand because the program, as we have heard, is simple but not easy. We pause on landings along the way: after the first three Steps (acceptance, hope, faith); after Steps Four through Seven (inner housecleaning); again after Eight and Nine (relationships with other people); and finally after the summing-up (Steps Ten, Eleven, and Twelve). We continue to make important discoveries about our inner selves, about how we relate to others, and about our spiritual links to a Higher Power.

We strive for progress, not perfection. We go back over the Steps again and again, understanding them a little better each time. We know, though, that we have the tools we need to transcend the emotional pain of our chronic illness. In the face of overwhelming odds, we move forward.

These are our own personal miracles, for which we are endlessly grateful.

CHAPTER THREE

Containing Your Hypertension

By practicing the principles of a Twelve Step program in your daily affairs, you will come to experience the serenity you need to manage your hypertension. You will know that you cannot cure yourself of hypertension but that you can minimize its harmful effects by working with your Higher Power. Above all, you will have learned to turn over the care of your disease to that Power.

Serenity doesn't mean apathy. Part of your responsibility to your Higher Power is to do all that is necessary to care for yourself. Your main goal is to contain your hypertension, to bring it under control quickly and permanently. This involves lifestyle changes. For most people, change is a challenge. Ask your Higher Power during daily prayer and meditation to give you the strength to change.

Avoiding the Easy Path

You also need to ask for the strength to avoid taking a path just because it's easy. Instead, ask for the strength to choose the path that is right for you.

The tendency is to believe that pharmaceuticals are the answer to all medical problems. Drug therapy is what most patients expect when first diagnosed with hypertension, and usually the first course of action doctors follow. Drug therapy for people with hypertension is costly and complex and may even be unnecessary in some cases. There are several ways for motivated people with hypertension to lower their blood pressure without using drugs. This is especially true in cases where the hypertension is mild and the causes of the condition appear obvious and manageable through lifestyle changes.

Take the example of a person with a blood pressure of 150/95 (a mildly elevated pressure). He is twenty pounds overweight, smokes, and rarely exercises. Drug therapy should be considered, but first, the patient can attempt to lower his blood pressure through a program that involves smoking cessation, exercise, and weight loss. In many cases, losing just ten pounds through diet and exercise is enough to return blood pressure to an appropriate level.

Some people who seem otherwise outwardly healthy have high blood pressure caused by excessive alcohol consumption. In fact, alcoholics with hypertension who abstain from alcohol for a period of time often see their blood pressure return to normal quickly—and, if they continue to remain sober, permanently. In addition, the stress associated with the life of an alcoholic frequently worsens hypertension. For alcoholics whose high blood pressure is caused by their drinking, complete abstention from alcohol is the absolute best hypertension therapy.

Alcohol and Hypertension

There is an established relationship between alcohol consumption and hypertension.

Consuming two or more drinks per day can cause blood pressure to rise from normal to high. Some patients diagnosed with primary hypertension have the condition because they are alcoholic. If alcoholics address their addiction by abstaining from alcohol, frequently their blood pressure returns to normal.

In some cases, if an active alcoholic does in fact have primary hypertension, abstaining from alcohol alone may not be enough to bring blood pressure down to a normal level, but it will enable a patient to take less extreme medical measures—including large amounts of antihypertensive medication—to get blood pressure under control.

The bottom line is that anyone who is an alcoholic needs to abstain from alcohol, and alcohol's ability to cause high blood pressure is just another reason why.

The Truth about Alcohol and Heart Health

You may have heard that some alcohol is good for your heart health. Indeed, some news reports suggest that people who consume a drink or two a day have lower blood pressure and live longer than those who consume excessive amounts of alcohol. Other reports note that wine raises the "good" blood cholesterol (HDL) which prevents the buildup of fats in the arteries. While these news stories may be correct, they don't tell the whole story: too much alcohol contributes to a host of other health problems, such as motor vehicle accidents, diseases of the liver and pancreas, damage to the brain and heart, an increased risk of many cancers, and fetal alcohol syndrome. Alcohol is also high in calories. So you should limit how much you drink. Individuals who are alcoholic or who think they might be alcoholic should disregard news information suggesting alcohol is "good for you."

Most often, a combination of behavior modification and appropriate drug therapy is necessary to bring high blood pressure under control. It is also important to commit to a program that addresses the emotional and spiritual challenges of your disease.

Behavior Modification

If certain correctable problems are causing or worsening your hypertension, then you must accept that you will have to commit to making several important lifestyle changes. Such changes are recommended health measures for all people but may be lifesavers for people with hypertension. These lifestyle changes will most likely be good for your hypertension, but they will also improve your life in ways you may not even imagine. Remember, the best way to get full satisfaction from life is to live the way you believe your Higher Power wants you to live.

Improve Diet

Diet in particular has been shown to have a major influence on blood pressure rates. People who are overweight, who consume large amounts of alcohol, and who eat food high in salt are at greater risk of hypertension. Obesity and alcoholism will be addressed separately. This section looks at how improving your diet can lower your blood pressure.

The diet shown to provide the greatest benefit to

people with high blood pressure is a "combination diet." This diet is rich in fruits, vegetables, and low-fat dairy products. It contains reduced amounts of saturated fat and very few foods high in salt, which is linked to high blood pressure.

These are some tips on how to create such a diet.

1. Cut back on how much meat you eat; when you do buy meat, be a health-smart shopper.

Limit your consumption of red meat, poultry, and seafood to six ounces a day. Although meat contains proteins and other nutrients that your body needs, it also has a lot of fat, calories, and cholesterol. Often people fill up on large portions of meat and don't eat enough vegetables and grains. You shouldn't eat more than two three-ounce servings a day; three or four ounces is about the size of a deck of cards.

- If you currently eat large portions of meat, cut back by one-half or one-third at each meal.
- Try to include two or more vegetarian-style meals every week.
- Include more servings of vegetables, rice, pasta, and beans so you need less meat to make a satisfying meal. Casseroles, pastas, and stir-fried dishes often include less meat and more vegetables, grains, and beans.

- Buy less meat. If it's not there, you won't eat it.
- Select lean cuts of red meat. "Lean" means low in fat. You can gauge how much fat there is in a piece of red meat by how much marbling there is in it. Choose cuts with the least amount of marbling, such as round or loin cuts.
- Follow a health-smart guide to grades of red meat. "Select meats" contain the least marbling and are lowest in fat and calories. "Choice meats" contain more fat and calories than select meats. "Prime meats" have the highest proportion of fat.
- Trim extra fat away. A key to getting lean protein from meat is to trim away visible fat. Trimming fat off a lean roast or chicken breast before you cook it prevents fat from "migrating" into the meat or poultry. Trimming reduces fat without reducing flavor.

2. Increase the amount of fruits and vegetables you eat.
   When planning meals, don't make meat the centerpiece of the meal. Think of red meat, poultry, and seafood as complements to fruits, vegetables, and dry peas and beans.

- If you eat only one or two servings of fruits and vegetables a day, add one serving at lunch and one at dinner.

- If you don't eat fruit or only have juice at break-fast, add fruit as a snack.
- Keep an abundance of brightly colored fresh fruit attractively displayed in your kitchen. It will be irresistible!

3. Lower your sodium intake.

Too much salt, or sodium, is a cause of high blood pressure. Most Americans eat much more salt than they need. Current recommendations are to consume no more than 2,400 milligrams a day of sodium—about one teaspoon of table salt. Few people add this much salt to their food at the table on a daily basis, yet they are getting it in their diet. How? Much of the salt we eat is added during food preparation, usually in fast foods or processed items.

Here are some tips to make sure you consume no more than 2,400 milligrams per day of sodium:

- One easy and effective way to cut back on salt is to simply remove the saltshaker from your table.
- Check food labels for sodium contents. Favor foods lower in sodium. Look for packaging that indicates the contents are low in sodium ("sodium free," "very low sodium," and so forth). Because they are usually very high in

salt, buy low- or reduced-sodium or "no-salt-added" versions of foods such as these:

—canned soup, dried soup mixes, bouillon
—canned vegetables and vegetable juices
—cheeses, lower in fat
—margarine
—condiments such as ketchup and soy sauce
—crackers and baked goods
—processed lean meats
—snack foods such as chips, pretzels, and nuts

• Buy fresh vegetables or ones that have been frozen or canned without salt added. Use fresh poultry, fish, and lean meat, rather than canned or processed types.
• Instead of adding salt when cooking, use herbs, spices, and salt-free seasoning blends.
• Don't add salt when cooking rice, pasta, and hot cereals. Avoid buying instant or flavored rice, pasta, and cereal mixes because they usually have added salt.
• Rinse canned foods such as tuna to remove some sodium.
• Choose "convenience" foods that are low in sodium. Cut back on frozen dinners, mixed dishes such as pizza, packaged mixes, canned

soups or broths, and salad dressings, which often
have a lot of sodium.

4. Choose dairy foods that are heart-healthy.

Dairy foods provide essential calcium and protein,
but they can also be high in saturated fat and cholesterol. Instead of full-fat dairy products, buy

- skim or 1-percent-fat milk
- nonfat or low-fat yogurt
- low-fat or fat-free ice cream and frozen yogurt
- reduced-fat, fat-free, or part-skim-milk cheeses
- low-fat or fat-free sour cream or cream cheese

5. Snack . . . but do it sensibly.

When you crave a snack, often it's a food characteristic such as crunchy, creamy, or cold that appeals
to you, not necessarily the food itself. Once you've
identified what you want, choose a health-smart food
that will satisfy your desire. Here are some ideas.

- Crunchy—reduced-fat or fat-free crackers, air-
  popped popcorn, raw vegetables, rice cakes,
  frozen grapes or strawberries
- Creamy or cold—nonfat frozen yogurt, fat-free
  ice cream, sorbet, juice bars, or fruit spritzers

Sodium in Foods (in milligrams)[1]

* Choices are higher in saturated fat, cholesterol, or both.

** Creamy soups are higher in saturated fat and cholesterol.

*** Limit main dishes that have ingredients higher in saturated fat, cholesterol, or both.

Meat, Poultry, Fish, and Shellfish

Fresh meat (including lean cuts of beef, pork, lamb, and veal), poultry, finfish, cooked, 3 oz. (less than 90)

Shellfish, 3 oz. (100–325)

Tuna, canned, 3 oz. (300)

* Sausage, 2 oz. (515)

* Bologna, 2 oz. (535)

* Frankfurter, 1 1/2 oz. (560)

Boiled ham, 2 oz. (750)

Lean ham, 3 oz. (1,025)

Eggs

Egg white, 1 (55)

* Whole egg, 1 (65)

Egg substitute, 1/4 cup = 1 egg (80–120)

---

1. Adapted from *Home and Garden Bulletin*, United States Department of Agriculture (July 1993): 253–57.

Dairy Products

Milk

* Whole milk, 1 cup (120)
Skim or 1-percent-fat milk, 1 cup (125)
Buttermilk (salt added), 1 cup (260)

Cheese

* Swiss cheese, 1 oz. (75)
* Cheddar cheese, 1 oz. (175)
* Blue cheese, 1 oz. (395)
Low-fat cheese, 1 oz. (150)
* Process cheese and cheese spreads, 1 oz. (340–450)
Lower-sodium and fat versions (read the label)
* Cottage cheese (regular), 1/2 cup (455)
Cottage cheese (low fat), 1/2 cup (460)

Yogurt

* Yogurt, whole milk, plain, 8 oz. (105)
Yogurt, fruited or flavored (low fat or nonfat), 8 oz. (120–150)
Yogurt, plain (nonfat or low fat), 8 oz. (160–175)

Vegetables

Fresh or frozen vegetables, or no-salt-added canned (cooked without salt), 1/2 cup (less than 70)

Vegetables, canned, no sauce, 1/2 cup (55–470)
* Vegetables, canned or frozen with sauce, 1/2
  cup (read the label)
Tomato juice, canned, 3/4 cup (660)

Breads, Cereals, Rice, Pasta, and Dry Peas and Beans

Breads and crackers

Bread, 1 slice (110–175)
English muffin, 1 (260)
Bagel, 1 (380)
Cracker, saltine type, 5 squares (195)
* Baking powder biscuit, 1 (305)

Cereals (Ready-to-eat)

Shredded wheat, 3/4 cup (less than 5)
Puffed wheat and rice cereals, 1 1/2 to 1 2/3 cup
(less than 5)
Granola-type cereals, 1/2 cup (5–25)
Ring and nugget cereals, 1 cup (170–310)
Flaked cereals, 2/3 to 1 cup (170–360)

Cereals (Cooked)

Cooked cereal (unsalted), 1/2 cup (less than 5)
Instant cooked cereal, 1 packet = 3/4 cup (180)

Pasta and rice

Cooked rice and pasta (unsalted), 1/2 cup (less than 10)
* Flavored rice mix, cooked, 1/2 cup (250–390)

Peas and beans

Peanut butter (unsalted), 2 tbsp. (less than 5)
Peanut butter, 2 tbsp. (150)
Dry beans, home cooked (unsalted) or no-salt-added canned, 1/2 cup (less than 5)
Dry beans, plain, canned, 1/2 cup (350–590)
* Dry beans, canned with added fat or meat, 1/2 cup (425–630)

Fruits

Fruits, fresh, frozen, canned, 1/2 cup (less than 10)

Fats and Oils

Oil, 1 tbsp. (0)
* Butter (unsalted), 1 tsp. (1)
* Butter (salted), 1 tsp. (25)
Margarine (unsalted), 1 tsp. (less than 5)
Margarine (salted), 1 tsp. (50)
Imitation mayonnaise, 1 tbsp. (75)
* Mayonnaise, 1 tbsp. (80)

Prepared salad dressing (low calorie), 2 tbsp.
(50–310)
* Prepared salad dressings, 2 tbsp. (210–440)

Snacks

Popcorn, chips, and nuts

Nuts (unsalted), 1/4 cup (less than 5)
Nuts (salted), 1/4 cup (185)
* Potato chips and corn chips (unsalted), 1 cup
  (less than 5)
* Potato chips and corn chips (salted), 1 cup
  (170–285)
Popcorn (unsalted), 2 1/2 cups (less than 10)
Popcorn (salted), 2 1/2 cups (330)

Candy

Jelly beans, 10 large (5)
* Milk chocolate bar, 1-oz. bar (25)

Frozen desserts

* Ice cream, 1/2 cup (35–50)
Frozen yogurt (low fat or nonfat), 1/2 cup
(40–55)
Ice milk, 1/2 cup (55–60)

Condiments

Mustard, chili sauce, hot sauce, 1 tsp. (35–65)
Ketchup, steak sauce, 1 tbsp. (100–230)
Salsa, tartar sauce, 2 tbsp. (85–205)
Salt, 1/6 tsp. (390)
Pickles, 5 slices (280–460)
Soy sauce (lower sodium), 1 tbsp. (600)
Soy sauce, 1 tbsp. (1,030)

Convenience Foods

** Canned and dehydrated soups, 1 cup (600–1,300)
** Lower-sodium versions (read the label)
*** Canned and frozen main dishes, 8 oz. (500–1,570)
*** Lower-sodium versions (read the label)

Lose Weight[2]

The more weight you carry around, the harder your heart has to pump. Being overweight can make you up to six times more likely to have high blood pressure than if you are the recommended weight for your body type. Losing just a few pounds can make the difference between having normal blood pressure or stage 1 hy-

2. The recommendations here do not take into consideration the special needs of people with dietary issues related to diabetes, wheat and sugar addiction, and other problems.

pertension. If you have stage 1 hypertension, losing a small amount of weight through diet and exercise may be enough to return your blood pressure to a healthy level. For those with more severe hypertension, weight loss in conjunction with medication is usually necessary to lower blood pressure.

Getting your weight to an appropriate level, then—and keeping it there—is an integral part of your program to get your blood pressure under control. How do you do this?

To lose weight you need to consume fewer calories than you burn. Don't rush it. That's because so-called crash diets trigger your body to hoard its fat reserves, and you'll regain the pounds you lost plus a few more. The healthiest and longest-lasting weight loss takes place when it occurs slowly—at a rate of about a half pound to one pound a week. You should never lose more than two and one-half pounds per week. For most people, cutting five hundred calories out of their daily diets and increasing their physical activity enables them to lose a pound every week.

To keep the weight off, you need to learn new eating habits that will last a lifetime. Most important, you need to change *what* you eat and *how much* you eat. Exercise is also crucial, and this will be covered in the next section of this chapter.

Changing What You Eat

An important part of losing weight is choosing foods low in calories and fat. Some common high-fat foods you should cut back on are fatty meats, poultry skin, butter, margarine, regular salad dressings, whole-milk dairy foods such as cheese, fried foods, and most cookies, cakes, and pastries. Foods rich in starch and fiber are excellent substitutes for high-fat foods. Such foods include fruits, vegetables, whole-grain cereals, pasta and rice, whole-grain breads, dry peas and beans. Most of these foods are also rich in vitamins and minerals.

Changing How Much You Eat

Weight loss doesn't depend just on what you eat—it also matters how much you eat. Most Americans simply eat too much. It's especially important to eat smaller portions of high-fat foods such as meats and cheeses. Restrict yourself to one moderate portion and don't go back for seconds. Getting acquainted with undesirable eating habits will help you do something about them. It might help to write down what you eat and when. So, for example, if you tend to snack on high-fat foods such as chocolate in the evenings when you watch television, you can make a point of substituting such foods with healthy, low-fat alternatives such as unbuttered, no-salt popcorn.

Increase Daily Physical Activity/ Begin an Exercise Program

Regular physical activity helps lower your blood pressure and helps you lose weight too, making it an important way to control hypertension. Physically active people are 20 to 50 percent less likely to develop high blood pressure than inactive people. In addition to lowering blood pressure, physical activity has other benefits: it reduces the risk of heart disease, lowers total cholesterol, and raises levels of the "good" HDL cholesterol.

Strenuous exercise isn't necessary—even moderate levels of physical activity, such as brisk walking and yard work, are beneficial. Try to work physical activity into your everyday life in simple ways like this:

- Use the stairs instead of the elevator/escalator.
- Get off the bus/subway one or two stops earlier and walk the rest of the way.
- Park farther away from the store or office.
- Work in the yard or garden.
- Go dancing.

For more on the benefits of exercise if you have high blood pressure, refer to chapter 5.

Exercise Guidelines

The following are some general guidelines for safe and successful exercise participation by people with hypertension.

- *Doc talk: If you have hypertension, it is absolutely essential that you speak with your doctor before starting an exercise program.*
- *Ease on in: Start off at a pace you can easily sustain; then increase the intensity of your program as you go on.*
- *Goal orientation: Set realistic but challenging goals for your exercise program. If you choose walking as your main form of exercise, increase the intensity of your walking program by following the table shown on page 107. Your ultimate goal is to work up to at least three moderate exercise sessions per week that each last between forty and seventy minutes.*
- *Decisions, decisions: Choose the right activity. Depending on the severity of your condition, certain sports may be beyond your capabilities. Walking is an excellent form of exercise for people with hypertension, and it can be done as a group social activity.*
- *Buddy up: Try to find a friend or two who will exercise with you. That way you'll motivate each other and you'll find yourself less likely*

to cancel a workout for fear of letting down
the other person.

- *Whose workout is it, anyway?:* Though it helps to get motivated by exercising with others, remember to set your own pace. You aren't competing against anyone but yourself. Let your exercise partners know how you feel.

- *Danger signs:* If you become nauseated or dizzy, weak, or short of breath, have palpitations, or experience pain, stop exercising immediately. You may want to consult your doctor, depending on the degree of pain or discomfort.

- *Cool it:* Take time to cool down after your workout. Slow down toward the end of your activity; then stretch for a few minutes after you stop.

- *Here's to you . . . :* When you achieve a goal— however modest—take time to congratulate yourself. Consider giving yourself a small reward. You deserve it!

Calories Burned during Physical Activities

* May vary depending on a number of factors including environmental conditions.

** Healthy man, 175 pounds; healthy woman, 140 pounds.

Activity	Calories Burned Up Per Hour*	
	Man**	Woman**
Light activity:	300	240
Cleaning house		
Playing baseball		
Playing golf		
Moderate activity:	460	370
Walking briskly (3.5 mph)		
Gardening		
Cycling (5.5 mph)		
Dancing		
Playing basketball		
Strenuous activity:	730	580
Jogging (9 min./mile)		
Playing football		
Swimming		
Very strenuous activity:	920	740
Running (7 min./mile)		
Racquetball		
Skiing		

Abstain from Alcohol

People who drink large amounts of alcohol on a regular basis are at greater risk of developing high blood pressure. Consuming three drinks a day can increase the flow of adrenaline (a hormone) to the point where it constricts blood vessels, which, in turn, raises blood pressure levels. Most hypertension resources advise people with high blood pressure to consume alcohol in moderation. However, such advice ignores the fact that the person who regularly drinks heavily is probably an alcoholic; for that reason, he or she needs to abstain completely from alcohol. One characteristic of alcoholism is that alcoholics are unable to control how much they drink—a characteristic which, leaving aside the other problems associated with alcoholism, has potentially lethal consequences for people with hypertension.

If you have high blood pressure and think you might be an active alcoholic, seek help through treatment or by attending a support group. Some alcoholics with high blood pressure who stop drinking see their blood pressure return to normal quite quickly. And if they continue to abstain, it remains at an appropriate level.

The nonalcoholic person with high blood pressure should follow standard recommendations advocating moderation in alcohol consumption. Limit how much alcohol you drink to no more than two drinks a day.

Manage Stress

There is a relationship between stress and hypertension. Although stress isn't a direct cause of primary hypertension, stress *does* increase blood pressure and is a concern for people who already have high blood pressure. As with alcohol, stress increases the body's flow of adrenaline, constricting blood vessels and raising blood pressure. For people with hypertension, stressful situations can raise blood pressure to dangerous levels that might precipitate a hypertensive crisis. You can benefit by learning skills to decrease the stress in your life and, whenever possible, by removing yourself from situations currently stressful to you.

One of the most effective ways to deal with stress is prayer. Praying evokes beneficial changes in the human body. These changes include decreases in blood pressure, heart rates, and breathing, all of which are characteristics of the "relaxation response" (see page 77). The relaxation response produces a spiritual feeling in about 25 percent of people—even the nonreligious— according to Herbert Benson, the Harvard Medical School doctor who first described it.

A short invocation known as the Serenity Prayer can be particularly effective. You can say it anytime you feel stress.

> God, grant me the serenity
> To accept the things I cannot change,
> The courage to change the things I can,
> And the wisdom to know the difference.

Following are some other ways to deal with stress:

- Exercise.
- Take time to relax with a good book, movie, or music.

- Develop new interests, or rekindle interests in past activities.
- Interact. Spend time with family and friends.
- Address a person or situation that's causing you stress.
- Join a support group.
- Learn about your disease, but don't obsess about it.

Relaxation and Stress Management Techniques

There are a variety of ways to evoke what is known as the "relaxation response"—a state in which you experience reduced muscle tension and lowered heart rate, metabolism, and blood pressure. The beauty of the relaxation response is that, with practice, you can return to this state at any time.

Among the most common relaxation techniques are "deep breathing" and "meditation."

Deep Breathing

Deep breathing is one of the simplest and most effective ways to relax. It's also practical because you can do it almost anywhere. Here is one breathing technique you can use.

- *Sit up straight or lie flat on your back.*
- *Breathe in slowly through your nose and*

imagine you are pushing that air deep into your belly.

- *Note how your belly expands as your lungs fill with air.*
- *Now breathe out slowly through your mouth.*
- *Continue breathing in this way, watching how your belly rises and falls.*
- *Do this twice a day for five minutes at a time.*

Meditation

Like deep breathing, meditation can be done almost anywhere, although most people prefer, and beginners may need, quiet and solitude. Meditation is a rest state. You actually rest more deeply when meditating than when sleeping. Generally, meditation can be classified as two different types: "concentrative" and "mindfulness" meditation.

In concentrative meditation you use a picture, a word or phrase (mantra), an object (such as a candle flame), or a sensation (such as breathing) to focus the mind. If your mind begins to wander, you refocus your attention on the item you have chosen.

Mindfulness meditation is more complicated. Instead of focusing on a single sensation or object, you allow thoughts, feelings, and images to float through your mind. You let these thoughts go in and out of your mind without expressing positive or negative feelings about them.

Find out more about meditation and other relaxation techniques by reading books on the subject or by taking classes. Discover which relaxation techniques work best for you and make them part of your day!

Stop Smoking

Smoking cigarettes increases the risk of developing cardiovascular disease, which can lead to high blood pressure. Smoking also reduces the effectiveness of high blood pressure medication and constricts blood vessels. Smokers who quit smoking, whatever their age, will reduce their risk of developing cardiovascular disease within one year.

A variety of options are available for people who want to stop smoking. Dozens of inpatient and outpatient smoking cessation programs exist around the country. Your doctor may be able to refer you to a program.

Nicotine replacement therapy may also play a useful role in smoking cessation. Forms of nicotine replacement include chewing gum, the patch, the inhaler, and pills. Research shows that these products work best when combined with some form of behavior therapy. Read up on the differences between the nicotine replacement therapies and talk to your physician about whether they are an advisable option for you.

The Twelve Steps can also serve as key tools to quitting smoking. Nicotine Anonymous (NA), a Twelve Step support group, can be the starting point for smokers trying to quit or can serve as continuing care for people who complete an inpatient or outpatient smoking cessation program. If there is no listing for Nicotine Anonymous in your local telephone book, check the organization's Internet site for a meeting close to where you live or work (www.na.org).

The Health Benefits of Quitting Smoking

If you haven't yet developed a serious, smoking-related medical condition, quitting has immediate and significant benefits.

Your circulation quickly improves and the deadly carbon monoxide levels in your blood start to decline. Your heart rate and blood pressure, which are unhealthily elevated by smoking, go down. Your senses of taste and smell come back within days, and breathing gets steadily easier.

In the long term, people who stop smoking live longer than those who continue with their cigarette habit. After ten to fifteen years, an ex-smoker's risk of an early death is approximately that of a person who has never smoked.

Stopping smoking dramatically lowers your chance of getting cancer, and this risk continues to decline the longer you stay "smoke-free." Lung cancer is the leading cause of cancer death, and the main risk factor for lung cancer is smoking cigarettes. After a person quits smoking, the risk of developing lung cancer gradually declines until, within ten years, the risk is 30 to 50 percent below that of a person who continues to smoke. The risk of contracting cancers of the mouth, throat, and esophagus lessens significantly by five years after quitting.

Smoking cessation will benefit you whatever your age. Some older men and women claim they don't feel the benefits of quitting. However, research shows that people sixty to sixty-four years old who quit smoking are 10 percent less likely to die during the next fifteen years than their peers who continue to smoke. Those who quit before age fifty experience even greater health rewards and their risk of dying in the next fifteen years is half that of smokers.

Medication for Hypertension

For some, lifestyle changes are enough to lower high blood pressure to appropriate levels. For others, medication is also needed. Remember that even if you need medication, you should continue your lifestyle changes. The improvements in your health will help the drug or drugs you take work better. Over time, the changes you have made in your lifestyle to correct issues such as weight and smoking may allow you to reduce the amount of medication you need to take.

Because no two people are exactly alike, anti-hypertensive drug therapy varies greatly. Your doctor will prescribe medication based on your medical condition.

Knowing Your Medications

Fortunately, there are many blood pressure drugs to-day. Although you may have to take the drug for a long time, you will get enormous health benefits from controlling your high blood pressure.

When the doctor prescribes a high blood pressure drug, be sure you understand the instructions. Know the dosage and the intervals at which you should take the medication.

If you are not sure about the instructions, ask while you are at the doctor's office or clinic. Write down the instructions. Later, if you do not remember something or are confused, call back and ask. Even if you are having the prescription filled and are unsure about the instructions, call. Do not be embarrassed. You cannot take the drug properly if you don't understand the instructions.

As with all drugs, those for high blood pressure can cause side effects. For example, some can make you sleepy or tired; others can cause a rash or cough.

Pay attention to how you feel. If you think you have an undesirable side effect, *do not stop taking the drug*. That can cause other problems. Instead, tell your doctor as soon as possible. The doctor will try to determine if the drug is the cause.

Once you begin a course of medications, the doctor will evaluate your progress within the first month of therapy. Some or all of the initial tests will be repeated and, based on the results, adjustments will be made to your medication type and dosage.

If the drug is causing a side effect, your doctor will probably change its dose or prescribe a different drug. It may take some adjustments to find the best dosage or drug for you.

Questions to Ask Your Doctor about Your Drug Therapy

Antihypertensive therapy can be complicated. Here are some questions to think about if your doctor has given you a prescription for anti-hypertensive medication.

- *Why has this drug been prescribed?*
- *How do I take it? With food? Without food? With other medications? Without other medications?*
- *What time of day should I take it?*
- *How many times a day should I take it?*
- *Will this new medication interact with any of the other medications I am taking? What kind of interactions are possible?*
- *What are the possible short- and long-term side effects?*
- *If I have side effects, what should I do?*
- *How does my doctor evaluate my progress after I begin therapy?*

Your doctor will reexamine you at regular intervals, usually starting within the first month of therapy, and will repeat some or all of the initial tests. He or she will then make any necessary adjustments to your prescription.

Compliance with Therapy

Even though you may not feel or have any symptoms due to hypertension, it is important that you take your medication. According to several studies, about half of the people with hypertension discontinue their medications within six months of starting. Ignoring your doctor's recommendations can lead to serious hypertension-related complications. These include worsening of coronary arteriosclerosis (hardening of the arteries), congestive heart failure, and kidney disease. In addition, noncompliance with medical advice can increase your chance of being admitted to the hospital for a hypertensive crisis if your blood pressure gets very high, very quickly. For all these reasons, it is extremely important to follow your doctor's instructions.

How High Blood Pressure Drugs Work

High blood pressure drugs work in various ways. They are designed to alter

- how hard the heart pumps
- how much the blood vessels widen and narrow
- how much fluid is in the body

Your doctor will choose the drug that best suits you. Often, two or more drugs work better than one drug.

The following are the main types of high blood pressure drugs:

- Diuretics: These are sometimes called water pills because they work in the kidneys and flush excess water and sodium from the body through urine. This reduces the amount of fluid in the blood. And, since sodium is flushed out of blood vessel walls, the vessels open wider, and blood pressure goes down. There are different types of diuretics. They are often used in conjunction with other high blood pressure drugs.

- Beta blockers: These reduce nerve impulses to the heart and blood vessels. This makes the heart beat less often and with less force. Blood pressure drops and the heart works less hard.
- Angiotensin antagonists: These are a new type of high blood pressure drug. They shield blood vessels from a hormone called angiotensin II, which normally causes vessels to narrow. As a result, the vessels open wider and pressure lowers.
- Angiotensin converting enzyme (ACE) inhibitors: These prevent angiotensin II from being formed. They relax blood vessels and pressure goes down.
- Calcium channel blockers (CCBs): These keep calcium from entering the muscle cells of the heart and blood vessels. Blood vessels relax and pressure goes down. Short-acting CCBs are taken several times a day. If you are on such a drug, you should talk with your doctor about other medication choices. The longer-acting types of CCB, which are taken once a day, do not produce these results.

- Alpha blockers: These work on the nervous system to relax blood vessels, which allows blood to pass more easily.
- Alpha-beta blockers: These work the same way as alpha blockers but also slow the heartbeat, as beta blockers do. As a result, less blood is pumped through the vessels.
- Nervous system inhibitors: These relax blood vessels by controlling nerve impulses.
- Vasodilators: These open blood vessels by relaxing the muscle in the vessel walls.

Confusion Associated with Hypertension Drug Therapy

The good news is that many drugs are available to treat hypertension. Detailed guidelines are available to help doctors make the right decisions regarding drug therapy for their patients. However, the sheer number and variety of these medicines can complicate drug therapy.

Depending on how the drugs are classified, eight or nine categories of high blood pressure drugs exist. Each category has several different drugs. In addition, each drug may have two or three different names. And don't forget that some hypertension drugs come in combination forms; that is, more than one drug is contained in an individual pill or capsule.

The drug treatment guidelines state factors that physicians must consider when prescribing hypertension medication. These factors include severity of high blood pressure, age, race, associated disease, drug interaction, and cost. Considering these factors gives physicians an opportunity to tailor treatment to the specific needs of individual patients.

It is extremely important, however, for patients to be vigilant about their drug therapy. You should not have reservations about questioning the doctor even before any problems occur.

Commitment to a Spiritual Program

Spirituality is your inherent belief in the existence of a Higher Power, energy, or force—which you may or may not choose to call God—and a feeling of closeness to that entity. If you have a chronic illness, spiritual belief will help you on two levels. One, it will help to heal you physically; and, two, it will show you how to develop the resolve you need to manage your disease.

Spirituality and Physical Healing

For more than twenty-five years, scientists at Harvard Medical School laboratories have systematically studied the benefits of mind-body interactions. Their research has established that prayer causes the body to experience a variety of healthful physiological changes, including lowered blood pressure. Regular prayer, meditation, or similar activity was shown to decrease the blood pressure of 80 percent of the people with hypertension studied; in 16 percent of the study group, blood pressure was reduced enough that participants were able to go off their medications.

Developing Coping Skills

A Twelve Step spiritual program shows that you have to accept you have hypertension before you can deal with the disease effectively. You turn over care of your disease to a Higher Power and dedicate yourself to cooperating with that Power. By following a Twelve Step program, you learn to work for your Higher Power, with your Higher Power, and through your Higher Power. Working the Steps has helped millions of people with chronic illnesses to effectively manage their disease.

Refer to the Twelve Steps for Hypertension on pages xxi–xxii.

CHAPTER FOUR

Women and Hypertension

Traditionally, hypertension has been regarded as a men's disease. It is now known that women are also candidates for high blood pressure. In fact, more women than men eventually develop hypertension. It is important for women to educate themselves about this silent killer so they can take steps to prevent and treat it in themselves.

The Age Factor

In young adulthood, high blood pressure is more common in men than women. Later in life, though, women with high blood pressure outnumber men and more women than men die of its effects. More than half of all women sixty-five and older have high blood pressure. In the United States, the highest incidences of hypertension are seen in black and Hispanic women.

Why do the rates of women with high blood pressure catch up to and eventually exceed the rates in men as they get older? There are three main reasons.

1. Before menopause, women benefit from the protective effects of estrogen, which keeps their arteries smoother and more flexible. With menopause, women stop producing estrogen and lose out on its protective effects. Thus, their likelihood of developing high blood pressure rises.
2. Both men and women are more likely to develop high blood pressure as they get older. But because women often live longer, there naturally will be more hypertensive women than men in the population.
3. A side effect of birth control pills can be high blood pressure.

Women, Race, and Hypertension

The distribution of hypertension in the female population differs according to race. Hypertension is more common, occurs earlier in life, and is more severe and less managed in black women than it is in women of other races. In all age groups up to seventy-five years old, the prevalence of high blood pressure is highest among black women, which puts them at the greatest risk of complications from hypertension. The prevalence of hypertension in Hispanic women is similar to that of white women up to age fifty-five. Thereafter, the prevalence of hypertension in Hispanic women is statistically in between that of white and black women. Asian women are least likely to develop hypertension.

Pregnancy and Hypertension

The relationship between pregnancy and hypertension is an issue for two reasons: (1) women with hypertension who get pregnant risk medical repercussions for mother and child, and (2) women with normal blood pressure who get pregnant may develop dangerous pregnancy-induced hypertension (preeclampsia).

Mothers with High Blood Pressure

Mothers with hypertension tend to have small placentas and their infants tend to be small at birth. The incidence of fetal death is also higher in these women than in the general population. A woman with hypertension who gets pregnant needs to be carefully monitored by her physician.

Pregnancy-Induced Hypertension (Preeclampsia)

Severe, sudden episodes of high blood pressure in pregnant women caused by a condition called pre-eclampsia can be very serious for both mother and child. The condition occurs in up to 10 percent of all pregnancies, usually in the third trimester of a first pregnancy, and goes away immediately after delivery.

The latest research shows that this condition may be

caused by a failure of the placenta to embed properly in the uterus, which causes it to misconnect with the mother's blood vessels. As a result, the fetus does not get enough blood supply and the mother's own blood pressure rises. Symptoms and signs of preeclampsia include protein in the urine and swollen ankles. The reduced supply of blood to the placenta can cause low birth weight and eye or brain damage in the fetus. Severe cases of preeclampsia can cause kidney damage, convulsion, and coma in the mother and can be lethal to both mother and child.

It is important that all expectant mothers, not just pregnant women with hypertension, have frequent examinations, blood and urine tests to determine whether their kidneys are functioning properly, and possibly repeat ultrasound exams to make sure the baby is growing properly.

Sometimes bed rest is necessary. In pregnant women whose blood pressure is very high, medication may be prescribed.

Effects of Birth Control Medication

Women who take the Pill are more likely to have high blood pressure than those who don't. A woman who is in the high range of normal blood pressure may see her blood pressure rise to a hypertensive level after she starts taking birth control pills. The Pill causes the kidneys to produce more of the blood-pressure-raising hormone renin. It can also cause weight gain and water retention, which are two more risk factors for high blood pressure.

Experts once thought that going off the Pill reduced the risk of hypertension. But a recent study shows that past use of the Pill caused elevated blood pressure in women into their seventies. If you are a woman thinking of taking the Pill, have your blood pressure checked beforehand. If you have high blood pressure, the Pill may not be a good birth control choice for you. If you do go on the Pill, have your blood pressure checked every six months.

Smoking and birth control pills are a particularly dangerous combination if you are prone to hypertension.

There are obviously unique aspects of hypertension in women—hypertension during pregnancy, for instance, and the effects of birth control pills on blood pressure. However, high blood pressure in women is currently treated in much the same way as it is in men. The key measures to controlling a woman's blood pressure are appropriate drug therapy and behavior modification (diet, weight control, exercise, stress management, smoking cessation, and abstaining from alcohol). It is also important to commit to a program that addresses the emotional and spiritual challenges of your disease.

Research is still being done to find out whether any specific risk factors for hypertension have a greater effect on women than men. For example, to assist in treatment and prevention it would help to know whether women's blood pressure is especially sensitive to salt consumption or increases in weight. Some things are known. For example, doctors know that birth control pills and smoking can cause extreme elevations in blood pressure in women. Another important area of research concerns whether women with hypertension respond better to any particular class of medication.

Hypertension and Heart-Lung Disease

Hypertension is one of the most important modifiable risk factors for cardiovascular (heart-lung) diseases such as stroke, heart attack, and congestive heart failure. Cardiovascular diseases kill more people than all other causes of death combined, including cancer. The death rate from heart-lung disease in men has decreased since the early 1980s, while the rate for women has increased and exceeded that of men since 1984. Heart attack has become the single-largest killer of both American men and women. Heart-lung disease kills nearly half a million women each year, more than ten times the number of deaths from either breast cancer or lung cancer. The statistics for black women are even more dire. Their mortality rate from heart attacks alone is about twice that of white women, and as many as 20 percent of all deaths in black women with hypertension can be attributed to high blood pressure.

Hypertension is also associated with stroke. Stroke claims the lives of approximately ninety thousand women each year. In 1992, women accounted for 61 percent of all deaths from stroke, and the death rate for black women was 77 percent higher than that for white women.

CHAPTER FIVE

Exercise to Control High Blood Pressure

For many people with hypertension, laziness is an obstacle to getting their blood pressure under control. If this is true for you, then in Step Seven of your Twelve Step program and during prayer and meditation, ask your Higher Power to remove this character defect so you can better manage your chronic disease.

Ridding yourself of laziness is especially important if you have hypertension. Exercise is an extremely effective weapon against primary hypertension. If you have stage 1, or mild, primary hypertension, endurance exercise such as running, aerobic dance, or swimming may be enough to reduce your blood pressure to satisfactory levels—and to keep it there if you continue exercising.[1] In fact, doctors are increasingly prescribing exercise as the sole initial treatment strategy for

1. A large number of studies have demonstrated that endurance exercise causes a 10 mm Hg average reduction in both systolic and diastolic blood pressures in persons with stage 1 primary hypertension (blood pressures 140–159/90–99 mm Hg).

people with stage 1 or 2 primary hypertension because it doesn't have the undesirable side effects of blood pressure medications. If you or your doctor chooses a physical fitness program as your sole course of therapy, have a follow-up blood pressure exam within a few weeks to make sure your exercise program is lowering your blood pressure; if it isn't, you may have to consider alternate therapies such as medication and diet.

An exercise program is also important if you have more severe high blood pressure. If you have stage 3 or 4 hypertension, you'll need to wait to begin an exercise program until you're on blood pressure medication and have discussed an exercise plan with your doctor.

The following pages contain the basic information you will need to begin and maintain a personal physical fitness program. You will learn what appropriate goals look like and how often, how long, and how hard you must exercise to achieve them. You will also find information that will make your workouts easier, safer, and more satisfying.

What Is Fitness?

The three main components of fitness are

- cardiovascular (heart and lung endurance): the ability of the heart and lungs to pump blood and deliver oxygen throughout the body

- muscle strength: the strength and endurance of your muscles
- joint flexibility: the ability to move your joints freely and without pain through a wide range of motion

If you have high blood pressure, the cardiovascular component of fitness is the most important. The types of exercise that improve heart-lung endurance are the ones most effective in lowering blood pressure. Furthermore, these activities usually help you lose weight, another important way to control blood pressure.

Exercises to improve strength and flexibility do help lower blood pressure, but not as effectively as heart-lung endurance activities. People with hypertension need to do more than stretch or work out with weights to control their blood pressure. However, there is definitely a place for strength and flexibility exercises in the workout program of someone with high blood pressure.

Fitness Fundamentals

The four most important aspects of your workout regimen are mode, frequency, duration, and intensity. These aspects refer to what kind of exercise you do, how often you exercise, how long you exercise, and how hard you exercise.

To lower blood pressure, it is recommended that

people with hypertension get the same quantity and quality exercise recommended to promote well-being in all healthy adults:

- mode: large muscle activities
- frequency: three to five times a week
- duration: twenty to sixty minutes
- intensity: 65 to 85 percent of maximum heart rate

Recent studies have shown that exercising at somewhat lower intensities—between 40 and 70 percent of maximum heart rate—appears to lower blood pressure as much as or more than exercising at higher intensities. This finding has special implications for the elderly and obese because of the increased tendency for intense exercise to cause heart problems and bone and joint injuries in these groups.

Mode

Participate in an activity that uses large muscle groups, can be done continuously, and is rhythmical in nature. Examples of such activities include walking or hiking, jogging, cycling or bicycling, cross-country skiing, aerobic dance, rope skipping, rowing, stair climbing, swimming, skating, and various endurance game activities such as squash, racquetball, or basketball.

Frequency

Get some form of exercise between three and five times a week.

If you exercise less than three times a week, you may not get adequate benefit. On the other hand, if you exercise more than five times a week, you will benefit only slightly more but will greatly increase the chance of injury. Spacing your workouts throughout the week—every other day, for instance—may give you the best results.

Duration

How long you exercise depends on how hard you plan to exercise, but a workout of between twenty and sixty minutes is usually recommended.

In addition to the time spent actually doing endurance exercise, you should also warm up for five to ten minutes and cool down for five to ten minutes afterward.

For developing heart-lung endurance, twenty to thirty minutes of jogging may be equivalent to forty or fifty minutes of walking. The actual number of minutes depends on your fitness level and on how fast you walk or jog. It's more strenuous for an unfit person to walk fast than it is for a fit person to jog slowly.

Until recently it was believed that exercise was beneficial to your health only if you kept your heart and lung rates pumping for twenty minutes continuously. It is now known that you can improve health by exercising in increments of ten minutes at a time, so long as the total adds up to more than thirty minutes a day.

Intensity

For someone with hypertension, exercising at a low or moderate intensity for a lengthy period is preferable to working out at a high intensity for a short amount of time.

Not only is it safer, but also it is an equally or more effective way to lower blood pressure. In addition, people tend to stick better with exercise programs that are of low to moderate intensity than they do with high-intensity programs.

One way to tell if you are working hard enough is by checking your heart rate. When you exercise, you should aim for a target heart rate that is between 65 and 85 percent of your maximum heart rate (remember, though, that decreases in blood pressure can be achieved by exercising at lower intensity levels, between 40 and 70 percent of maximum heart rate).

A good guideline is that you should be able to carry on a conversation while exercising. This is the so-called talk test.

Your target heart rate can best be determined by a

medical or exercise professional. However, you can estimate your heart rate target yourself. First, calculate your approximate maximum heart rate by taking 220 and subtracting your age. Multiply this number by 0.50. This will be your minimum heart rate for exercising. The maximum exercise level will be 0.85 of your maximum heart rate. For example: A thirty-two-year-old man would have a maximum heart rate of 188 (220-32=188). He would have a target heart rate range of 94 to 160 beats per minute (188 x 0.50 = 94; 188 x 0.85 = 160; therefore, the range is 94–160). Bear in mind that maximum heart rate decreases with age and varies considerably at all ages, as much as twenty-five beats per minute or more. Therefore, to get a precise target heart rate you should consult a physician or a certified exercise professional and take an exercise test.

A Walking Program for People with Chronic Obstructive Pulmonary Disease (COPD)

The walking program described here is designed for people who haven't exercised for some time. Even if you are very unfit, you can do the walking sessions described in the early part of the program. Each walk session is divided into three parts: the warm-up phase, the target zone phase, and the cool-down phase. Of these three phases, the target zone requires explanation.

Achieving the Target Zone

To get the maximum benefit from exercise, it is necessary to exercise hard enough that your heart and lungs are working at between 65 and 85 percent of their maximum capabilities.

To check to see if you're exercising within your target zone, you need to take your pulse while you're exercising. Here's how:

- *Place the tips of your fingers over one of the major blood vessels (try just to the left or right of your Adam's apple or the spot on the inside of your wrist below the bone of your thumb).*
- *Count the number of times your heart beats during a ten-second period. Then multiply that number by six to figure out how many times a minute your heart is beating.*
- *Compare your heart rate with the chart below. For instance, if you are sixty-five years old, your goal is to have a target zone between 78 and 116 beats per minute.*

Age	Target Heart Rate Zone
20 years	100–150 beats per minute
25 years	98–146 beats per minute
30 years	95–142 beats per minute
35 years	93–138 beats per minute

Age	Target Heart Rate Zone
40 years	90–135 beats per minute
45 years	88–131 beats per minute
50 years	85–127 beats per minute
55 years	83–123 beats per minute
60 years	80–120 beats per minute
65 years	78–116 beats per minute
70 years	75–113 beats per minute

	Warm-Up Phase	Target Zone Phase	Cool-Down Phase	Total
Week 1				
Session A	Walk normally, 5 min.	Walk fast, 5 min.	Walk normally, 5 min.	15 min.
Session B	repeat	repeat	repeat	repeat
Session C	repeat	repeat	repeat	repeat

Each week do the walking session three times, as shown above for week one. If you find you reach a point where the sessions leave you overly fatigued (tired enough that you don't think you could go to the next level), repeat that week's program until you think you are fit enough to move on to the next level. It isn't necessary for you to complete the program in twelve weeks.

	Warm-Up Phase	Target Zone Phase	Cool-Down Phase	Total
Week 2	Walk normally, 5 min.	Walk fast, 7 min.	Walk normally, 5 min.	17 min.
Week 3	Walk normally, 5 min.	Walk fast, 9 min.	Walk normally, 5 min.	19 min.
Week 4	Walk normally, 5 min.	Walk fast, 11 min.	Walk normally, 5 min.	21 min.
Week 5	Walk normally, 5 min.	Walk fast, 13 min.	Walk normally, 5 min.	23 min.
Week 6	Walk normally, 5 min.	Walk fast, 15 min.	Walk normally, 5 min.	25 min.
Week 7	Walk normally, 5 min.	Walk fast, 18 min.	Walk normally, 5 min.	28 min.
Week 8	Walk normally, 5 min.	Walk fast, 20 min.	Walk normally, 5 min.	30 min.
Week 9	Walk normally, 5 min.	Walk fast, 23 min.	Walk normally, 5 min.	33 min.

	Warm-Up Phase	Target Zone Phase	Cool-Down Phase	Total
Week 10	Walk normally, 5 min.	Walk fast, 26 min.	Walk normally, 5 min.	36 min.
Week 11	Walk normally, 5 min.	Walk fast, 28 min.	Walk normally, 5 min.	38 min.
Week 12	Walk normally, 5 min.	Walk fast, 30 min.	Walk normally, 5 min.	40 min.

Week 13 onwards: Remember to check your pulse periodically during the target zone phase to make sure you are exercising in that zone. As your lungs adapt to the demands of this walking program, try exercising in the upper range of your target zone. Gradually increase your fast-walking time to between thirty and sixty minutes three or four times a week. With a five-minute warm-up and cool-down period, your walking sessions should last forty to seventy minutes.

Beneficial Effects of Exercise on Hypertension

Exercise has the following effects on hypertension:

- *reduces severity of primary hypertension*
- *reduces severity of secondary hypertension caused by renal dysfunction*
- *prevents or significantly slows down the onset of hypertension in at-risk people and reduces its severity if and when the disease develops*
- *significantly reduces the risk of an early death even when blood pressure does not lower (people who exercise but continue to have hypertension are much less likely to die from related illnesses than people with hypertension who are inactive and unfit; in some studies, people with hypertension who exercise regularly have lived longer than sedentary people with normal blood pressure)*

Maintaining Fitness and Lowered Blood Pressure

Blood pressure improves quickly in response to exercise. However, to keep your blood pressure level down you need to exercise regularly. You can miss a workout occasionally and it shouldn't affect your fitness or blood pressure levels, just so long as you don't stop working out altogether. You will begin to see a decline in your fitness and a rise in blood pressure after just two weeks of missing workouts and will probably be back to your original level of unfitness and pre-exercise blood pressure within three to five months.

Exercise requires a lifelong commitment of time and effort. Exercise must be a part of your daily life, like bathing and brushing your teeth.

Exercising for Weight Loss

Being overweight is a major risk factor for hypertension. That is in part why exercise—which can help you lose weight—is important to anyone trying to control his or her high blood pressure.

The goal of a weight loss program for someone with hypertension is to reduce body fat. To lose body fat you might need to exercise five days a week for a minimum of thirty minutes per session. People with hypertension should avoid short bursts of intense exercise.

Exercise together with diet is the most effective way to lose weight. Exercise itself may have only a modest effect on weight (unless you are severely obese and have not exercised for a long time). Diet has an especially important role for people with high blood pressure, as seen in chapter 3, Containing Your Hypertension (see pages 53–89). Diets that promise weight loss without exercise usually cause an undesirable loss of muscle as well as fat. Exercise helps maintain muscle and bone mass. Strength training with weights can be an extremely effective way of increasing the ratio of lean muscle mass to body fat.

The Importance of Flexibility Exercises and Strength Training

A well-rounded fitness program also includes workouts to improve strength and flexibility. Stretching and strengthening exercises have special implications for people with high blood pressure.

Flexibility Exercises

The safest and most effective way to develop flexibility is with static stretching, during which you stretch a muscle to the point of tension and then hold that position. Remember to breathe while you're holding the stretch. Done properly, a static stretching program can help lower blood pressure because it relaxes you. Many good books on stretching can be found in your local bookstore or library.

Strength Training

Free weights, strength-training machines, and calisthenics are all effective ways to build strength. Strength training has been shown to help reduce resting blood pressure.

Until quite recently, however, it was believed that strength training was risky for people with high blood pressure. Lifting weights, it was thought, would actually raise blood pressure. This incorrect conclusion was reached by testing professional weight lifters, many of whom abused anabolic steroids (which can raise blood pressure) to "bulk up." When done properly, strength training with weights lowers blood pressure by causing blood vessels to widen. In addition, if you work out with weights, you won't strain as much when doing chores such as carrying groceries, an activity that can cause already-high blood pressure to rise to dangerous levels.

Strength training may have special implications for seniors with hypertension. As people age, they lose muscle mass. The relative rise in body fat that occurs during this process is linked to the onset of high blood pressure. Strength training exercises, however, can slow or reverse this process, even in the very elderly, leading to improvements in blood pressure levels.

Strength training should not be your sole form of antihypertensive exercise therapy, but it is an important part of an all-round fitness program to improve

Do	Don't
isotonic exercises, wherein the muscles change length, typified by lifting a dumbbell	do isometric exercises, exemplified by pushing against an immobile object such as a door frame, as this can raise blood pressure

Do	Don't
lift light or moderate-sized weights many times (between eight and fifteen repetitions)	lift very heavy weights just a few times
breathe in while you lift the weight, and breathe out while you return to the starting position	hold your breath while you lift the weight
move relatively quickly from one strength-training exercise to the next (known as circuit training).	Take long breaks between sets of exercises

Table 5.1. Strength Training for
People with Hypertension

your condition. As table 5.1 shows, if you have hypertension, there are do's and don'ts for working out with weights.

In fact, the guidelines for strength training if you have high blood pressure are virtually the same as for anyone else—only it's more important for people with hypertension to observe these guidelines. A qualified personal trainer will be able to advise you on how to work out properly with weights.

The following are some other important strength-training recommendations:

- Do strength training at least twice but not more than three times per week. If you are not interested in large strength gains, you can get almost as much improvement (70 to 80 percent as much) by doing strength training two times a week instead of three.
- Include eight to ten exercises that use major muscle groups in both the upper and lower body (arms, shoulders, chest, abdomen, back, hips, and legs).
- Do at least one set of each exercise, and no more than three.
- Each set should consist of eight to fifteen repetitions, which should nearly exhaust the muscle group being exercised.
- Make your strength-training session last between twenty and fifty minutes.
- Do the exercise through the full range of movement and don't jerk or overly strain to lift the weight.

One of the principal reasons for the rise in hypertension and other chronic diseases in Western society is the decline of physical activity. Many people no longer live the kinds of lives that provide sufficient physical activity. If you fall into that category, you need to look for other ways to get your necessary exercise.

A few generations ago, Americans did not need to jog or do aerobics. People got plenty of exercise in daily life. They tilled fields and stoked the furnaces of industry using old-fashioned muscle power. In 1850, human muscle provided nearly one-third of the energy used in workshops and factories and on farms. Today the comparable figure is less than 1 percent. But the human body's muscular, respiratory, and circulatory systems have not changed. They were designed for— and require—regular and vigorous use.

Whenever you feel like skipping a workout, ask your Higher Power to give you the resolve you need to put on your sweats and sneakers and get on with it. Remember, the best way to get full satisfaction from life is to live the way you believe your Higher Power wants you to live.

CHAPTER SIX

Complementary and Alternative Treatments for Hypertension

You have turned over control of your disease to a Higher Power. In doing so you have agreed to do your part in taking care of yourself. That includes finding out what treatments are available that may help alleviate or improve your condition, even those treatments outside the realm of conventional medicine.

Complementary and alternative medicines are treatments and health care approaches not taught widely in Western medical schools, not generally used in hospitals, and not usually reimbursed by medical insurance. The term covers a wide range of ancient healing philosophies, approaches, and therapies.

The terms "alternative" and "complementary" are both used because some of these therapies are used instead of conventional medicine ("alternative"), and others are used in conjunction with conventional medicine ("complementary").

Certain complementary and alternative approaches are based on familiar principles of Western medicine, but many have quite different origins. Many therapies remain far outside the realm of accepted Western medicine, while others have been embraced by large segments of society.

Consider, for instance, the ancient Chinese medical practice of acupuncture. Once considered quite bizarre in the West, it is now increasingly used by ordinary Americans to treat common medical conditions, to relieve stress, and even to ease symptoms during nicotine withdrawal. The same is true for herbal medicine, as evidenced by the television commercials for products containing echinacia, ginseng, and Saint-John's-wort. Given their increasing popularity among those attracted by low cost, lack of side effects, and purported effectiveness, many forms of medicine presently considered offbeat will eventually become accepted by mainstream health culture.

It is a measure of society's interest in alternatives to conventional medicine that in 1992 the government-run National Institutes of Health (NIH) created the Office of Alternative Medicine (OAM). OAM facilitates research and evaluation of unconventional medical practices and disseminates this information to the public. Its budget in 1998 was $20 million. You can obtain a classification of forty-seven complementary and alternative medical health care practices from the OAM. The list is intended to show the diversity of the field and is neither complete nor authoritative.

Many practitioners of conventional health care continue to dispute the claims of alternative and complementary medicine. That is because, by and large, such therapies are not investigated using the same scientific research methods used in conventional medicine. The benefits of such treatments, Western-trained doctors argue, are strictly anecdotal; that is, based on patient testimonials, not documented results. It is unlikely that alternative and complementary medicine will be fully accepted until its practitioners can produce results based on systematic, explicit, and comprehensive knowledge and skills.

How to Find Out More about Complementary and Alternative Treatments for Hypertension

Health care providers are becoming more familiar with alternative and complementary treatments, and your doctor may be willing to refer you to such a practitioner. The medical profession, however, is by and large suspicious of medical treatment it considers untested, unproved, and potentially harmful.

Don't be discouraged if your doctor cannot or will not provide you with the information you want. Information about particular complementary and alternative medical practices is available on the Internet and in medical libraries, public libraries, and popular bookstores.

Other resources for information are the NIH's twenty-four institutes, centers, and divisions. For information from the NIH on hypertension itself, call (301) 496-4000 and ask the operator to direct you to the appropriate office.

The advent of the Internet has made research into alternative and complementary medicine much easier—especially for people with chronic illnesses such as hypertension whose mobility is restricted. If you have a telephone line and can afford a computer, then the vast resources of the Internet are available to you. If you can't afford a computer, you should be aware that many libraries have computers that are hooked up to the Internet for use by library members. Once you are online, access to most medical research resources on the Internet is free. Some sites—such as thriveonline.com—take the latest medical research and "translate" it into information the ordinary person can understand. An excellent online source of complementary and alternative medicine is the alternative medicine section of www.healthanswers.com. Lessons in the basics of using the Internet are widely available, and classes may be held at your local library, senior center, or adult learning center.

To find out more about complementary and alternative treatments for hypertension, you may also want to ask practitioners of complementary and alternative medicine about their practices. Many practitioners belong to a growing number of professional associations, educational organizations, and research institutions that provide information about complementary and alternative medical practices. A growing number of these organizations have sites on the Internet that can easily be found.

Be aware that some of these organizations advocate a specific therapy or treatment but are unable to provide complete and objective health information.

How to Find a Practitioner in Your Area

To find a qualified complementary and/or alternative medical health care practitioner, contact medical regulatory and licensing agencies in your state (your health care provider should be able to provide you with their names). Such regulatory and licensing bodies can provide information about a specific practitioner's credentials and background. Many states license practitioners who provide alternative therapies such as acupuncture, chiropractic services, and massage therapy.

You also may locate individual practitioners by asking your health care provider or by contacting a professional association or organization. These organizations can provide names of local practitioners and information about how to determine the quality of a specific practitioner's services.

What to Consider When Choosing an Alternative Health Therapy or Practitioner

The health decisions you make are important, and choosing to explore complementary and alternative treatments is no exception. There are some serious issues you need to address when selecting an alternative or complementary therapy or practitioner. In particular, ask yourself questions about safety and effectiveness of the treatment, the qualifications of the practitioner, and the cost of the therapy.

Is It Safe? Is It Effective?

The therapy should provide relief from the condition for which it is sought—in this case, hypertension—and it should not have the ability to cause you harm when used as intended. Unfortunately, less is known about the safety and effectiveness of complementary and alternative products and practices than conventional medicine. So what can you do?

Ask the alternative/complementary health practitioner for evidence of the safety and effectiveness of the practice, treatment, or technology he or she advocates. Request information on new research that either supports or debunks the effectiveness of the treatment, and also ask about any new information about its safety.

You should also ask questions about possible side effects, interactions with other medications you are taking, expected results, and how long the treatment should last.

Make sure the practitioner is aware of all other therapies—both conventional and alternative/complementary—you are using, as this information will probably be necessary to ensure the safety and effectiveness of the treatment plan.

Published information on the safety and effectiveness of particular therapies can be found in scientific journals available at certain public libraries, university libraries, medical libraries, online computer services, and the U.S. National Library of Medicine (NLM) at the NIH. As the articles in these journals can be difficult for the layperson to understand, you might find the summary at the beginning of the manuscript, known as the "abstract," the easiest way to gain information from these materials. You can find these scientific articles in the *Index Medicus*, a published resource available in medical and university libraries and some public libraries.

The World Wide Web can be an excellent source of

information about the safety and effectiveness of complementary and alternative medicine, although it is important that you learn to differentiate between credible and noncredible sources. This ability to discern comes with time spent using the Internet.

Also try to gain access to people with hypertension who have received the treatment you are researching. Remember, though, that anecdotal evidence from other patients is not an accurate measure of the safety and effectiveness of a treatment. Therefore, it should not be the sole criteria for selecting an alternative or complementary therapy. Studies done under controlled conditions by trained medical scientists are the best way to assess a treatment's effectiveness.

What Are the Practitioner's Qualifications?

Research the background, qualifications, and reputation of the practitioner. You can do this by contacting the state or local regulatory body that has jurisdiction over the practice of the therapy you are seeking. Although complementary and alternative medicine is not as strictly regulated as conventional medicine, licensing and accreditation are continually being introduced.

Local and state medical boards may be able to provide information about an individual practitioner's credentials, and consumer affairs departments such as the Better Business Bureau can tell you whether there have been any complaints lodged against that person.

How Much Does It Cost?

Your health insurer or the practitioner should be able to tell you whether a particular therapy is covered by insurance. However, most complementary and alternative treatments are not covered by health insurance. Patients usually have to pay the entire amount of the therapy. Thus, cost is a very important factor for people seeking alternate and complementary medical treatment.

"Shop around" to find out what different practitioners charge for the same service. Although cost shouldn't be the sole criterion for selection, knowing what a variety of practitioners charge will give you some idea of what is appropriate. The same professional and regulatory bodies that can provide information on safety and effectiveness should be able to provide approximate cost guidelines.

Specific Alternative/Complementary Treatments for Hypertension

Several specific forms of alternative and complementary treatments are commonly used to treat hypertension. Some of these modalities—including acupressure, acupuncture, massage, and yoga—work by helping you relax.

During the last thirty years the most exciting development in the field of alternative and complementary medicine to treat hypertension has been the study of the mind's capacity to affect the body, or mind-body medicine. More work needs to be done, but there is a growing body of evidence that mind-body therapies, if appropriately selected and wisely applied, are a safe, effective, and inexpensive way to treat a variety of medical conditions, including hypertension. Specific mind-body interventions include psychotherapy, imagery, hypnosis, biofeedback, dance therapy, music therapy, art therapy, meditation, support groups, and prayer. Of these, biofeedback, imagery, meditation, and prayer are considered among the most effective in lowering blood pressure.

Biofeedback

Biofeedback uses computerized machines to measure and display body functions such as blood pressure, heart rate, skin temperature, muscle tension, and brain activity. By watching the monitoring device, you can learn by trial and error to adjust your thinking and other mental processes in order to control these bodily functions. In time, you will be able to lower your blood pressure alone and without the need for feedback from machines.

Imagery

Imagery involves using your imagination to effect physiological reactions. Simple and straightforward imagery—such as picturing yourself floating calmly in a lake—can help reduce your blood pressure. Here is a slightly more involved imagery exercise to lower blood pressure: Picture yourself going to the refrigerator and taking out three or four ice cubes. Imagine slowly washing your head, neck, and face with the ice cubes. Feel the coolness going into your skin, then going into your bloodstream, and then going to your brain. Sense an icy feeling taking over your body, starting in the neck and torso, then entering your arms and legs. At that time, envision that your blood pressure is within a normal range.

Prayer and Meditation

For more than twenty-five years, scientists have systematically studied the effects of prayer and meditation on high blood pressure. Their research has established that such activity causes the body to experience a variety of healthful physiological changes, including lowered blood pressure. The Twelve Steps described in detail in chapter 2 emphasize the importance of prayer and meditation for achieving spiritual health. Scientists have demonstrated in controlled studies that prayer and meditation also help improve physical health by, among other things, lowering blood pressure. The ability of prayer and meditation to do this reinforces the potential benefit of the Twelve Steps for anyone with a chronic illness.

However, alternate or complementary treatments should not be a substitute for any hypertension treatments prescribed by your doctor. Before you use an alternative or complementary treatment, carefully discuss this decision with your doctor.

Benefits of Meditation

Studies have found that regular meditation does the following:

- *reduces blood pressure*
- *reduces chronic pain*
- *reduces anxiety*
- *reduces serum cholesterol level*
- *reduces substance abuse*
- *increases intelligence-related measures*
- *reduces post-traumatic stress syndrome*
- *increases longevity and quality of life*
- *lowers health care costs*

Yoga Exercises for High Blood Pressure

Yoga is an ancient Indian system of exercises done to promote self-control of the body and mind. Experts say yoga offers specific exercises and techniques you can do yourself to help lower high blood pressure. Two yoga poses—the "horizontal healer" and the "knee squeeze"—are especially useful for people with high blood pressure because they improve circulation and relieve tension.

The Horizontal Healer: Lie on your back on the floor (use an exercise mat if you find it more comfortable), your arms at your sides, palms facing up. Your legs should be straight, your feet in a relaxed position. Close your eyes, relax all your muscles, and hold the pose for thirty seconds to several minutes, until your muscles completely relax. Breathe deeply. Mentally scan your body for any tension. If you feel tension anywhere, concentrate on the area in such a way as to relax the muscles. Note: If you feel pain in your lower back, keep your knees bent while doing this exercise.

The Knee Squeeze: Lie faceup on the floor or on an exercise mat, hands at your sides, toes slightly pointed.

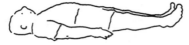

Inhale slowly and fully as you raise your right knee to your chest. Using both arms, hold the knee to your chest for a few seconds.

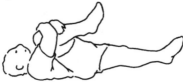

Then exhale as you straighten your knee and return your leg slowly to the starting position on the floor.

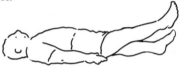

Do the same with your left leg. Repeat three times with each leg. Next breathe in deeply and then lift both knees to your chest at the same time.

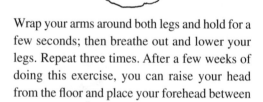

Wrap your arms around both legs and hold for a few seconds; then breathe out and lower your legs. Repeat three times. After a few weeks of doing this exercise, you can raise your head from the floor and place your forehead between your knees as far as possible.

Several yoga instructional books are available in stores. Choose two other exercises in addition to the ones described above to improve your circulation and to relieve tension. However, do not do inverted positions such as the headstand, as such positions can dangerously elevate high blood pressure.

Appendix

The following organizations can provide further information about the prevention, causes, and treatment of hypertension. In no way is this intended to be a complete or comprehensive list. The contact details were correct at the time of publication.

National Heart, Lung, and Blood Institute (NHLBI)

The NHLBI is part of the federal government's National Institutes of Health and provides a vast amount of information about research into hypertension and other related diseases.

The office is open during regular business hours to accept orders for publications and to provide information on the prevention and treatment of heart, lung, and blood diseases, including high blood pressure. As a research institute, the NHLBI does not provide referrals to doctors or counsel people on specific medical problems.

Phone: (301) 592-8573
Fax: (301) 592-8563

```
Internet:   www.nhlbi.nih.gov
E-mail:     NHLBIinfo@rover.nhlbi.nih.gov
Mail:       NHLBI Information Center
            Attention: Web Site
            P.O. Box 30105
            Bethesda, MD 20824-0105
```

The Framingham Heart Study

The Framingham Heart Study is renowned for its advances in the study of heart disease and hypertension. This group is affiliated with the National Heart, Lung, and Blood Institute, but as a research group, it is more likely to offer "cutting-edge" information.

```
Phone:      (508) 872-6562
Internet:   www.framingham.com
E-mail:     sandra@fram.nhlbi.nih.gov
```

American Heart Association (AHA)

The AHA is one of the world's premier health organizations. It has 2,000 state and metropolitan affiliates, divisions, and branches throughout the United States and Puerto Rico. Call the main number to locate the office nearest you. The AHA's Internet site has a section with an extensive amount of information about hypertension.

Phone: 800-AHA-USA1
Internet: www.amhrt.org

Doctor's Guide to Hypertension Information and Resources

This is an Internet site that provides an extensive amount of the latest legitimate medical news for patients or friends and relatives of patients diagnosed with hypertension and hypertension-related disorders.

Internet: www.pslgroup.com/
           hypertension.htm

Dietary Approaches to Stop Hypertension (DASH) Study Group

This is a group of Harvard doctors who have developed an effective, user-friendly diet that lowers high blood pressure. The diet is strongly endorsed by the National Heart, Lung, and Blood Institute and the American Heart Association. Easy-to-use guidelines for following the diet are available on the DASH Web site.

Internet: dash.bwh.harvard.edu

Index

A

acceptance, vii–viii, 23, 41–42
  of alternative therapies, 118, 119
  of Higher Power, 22
  of hypertension, x, xx, 17, 57, 89
  of self, 31, 32, 33–34, 36, 44
  of Twelve Step programs, xviii
acupressure, 125
acupuncture, 118, 121, 125
adrenal gland tumors, 7
adrenaline, 74, 75–76
African people. *See* black people

age factors, 9, 91–93, 105
  in exercising, 106–7, 113
AHA (American Heart Association), 132, 133
alcohol consumption, 16, 40, 54–57, 74–75
  and blood pressure readings, 13
  and heart health, 56–57
  as risk factor, 1, 7, 54–55, 74
alcoholics. *See* substance abuse
Alcoholics Anonymous, vii, ix, xix–xx
  Twelve Step program for, xxii–xxiii

alpha blockers, 87
alternative therapies, xv,
    117–30
    for hypertension,
        125–30
    insurance coverage
        for, 117, 125
    practitioners of,
        121–25
    resistance to, 118, 119
    safety/effectiveness
        of, 122–24
amends, 40–44
    indirect, 42–43
    to ourselves, 41, 44
American Heart
    Association (AHA), 9,
    132, 133
American Medical
    Association, xii
anger, xii, 17, 36, 44–45
angina, 3–4, 19
angiotensin antagonists,
    86
antihypertensive therapy.
    See medications

anxiety, 17, 34–35,
    128
apologies. *See* amends
arteries
    and estrogen, 92
    renal, 7
    See also hearts
arteriosclerosis, 3, 85
art therapy, 126
Asian people, 5, 93

B

Benson, Herbert, 76
beta blockers, 86
Better Business Bureau,
    124
biofeedback, 126
birth control pills, 7, 16,
    92, 94–95
    and smoking, 95, 96
black people, 5, 6, 8–9
    and gender factors, 9,
        91, 92–93, 97
blood, 1, 2, 7
    carbon monoxide lev-
        els in, 80

circulation of, 80,
128–30
clotting of, 4
oxygen in, 3, 100
blood pressure, 1, 2–3
readings of, 10,
11–13, 14
blood vessels, 18–19,
75–76
medication effects on,
85–87
and preeclampsia, 94
and smoking, 79
body fat, 111, 113
body fluids, 85–86, 95
brain functions, ix, 4, 18,
94, 126
breast cancer, 96–97
breathing exercises,
77–78

C

calcium channel blockers
(CCBs), 86
calories, 56, 69, 70,
73–74

in meats, 58, 59
cancer, 81, 96–97
cardiovascular system,
96–97, 100–101
character defects, 31, 32,
37–38, 44–45
and chronic illness,
33, 37, 99
chest pain, 3–4, 11, 19
children, 9–10, 93–94
Chinese medical prac-
tices, 118
chiropractic services,
121
cholesterol, 3, 58, 62, 63
HDL, 56, 71
chronic illness, xi–xii
from addiction, vii, xii
and character defects,
33, 37, 99
denial of, viii
emotional pain of, 17,
27–28, 35, 36, 44,
51
management of, xvii,
24–25, 44, 48

by admitting health problems, 24, 27
with positive feelings, 44, 45
through spirituality, xv, xvi, 17–18, 25–29, 45–46, 88
clergy, 31–32, 35
complementary therapies, xv, 117–30
for hypertension, 125–30
insurance coverage for, 117, 125
practitioners of, 121–25
resistance to, 118, 119
safety/effectiveness of, 122–24
convenience foods, 61–62
counselors, 31–32, 35
courage, 25, 31, 33, 43, 45
crash diets, 69

D
dairy products, 5, 58, 62, 64
dance therapy, 126
denial, viii, x, xx, 48
diabetes, viii
diastolic pressure, 2–3, 11, 12, 13
diet, 1, 5, 16, 54, 57–70
DASH, 133
and exercise, 111
and weight loss, 68–70
Dietary Approaches to Stop Hypertension (DASH) Study Group, 133
diuretics, 85–86
dizziness, 11, 73
Doctor's Guide to Hypertension Information and Resources, 133
drug therapy. *See* medications

E
eating habits, 69–70

echinacea, 118
Eighth Step, xxi, xxiii, 39–42, 44
Eleventh Step, xxii, xxiii, 45–46
e-mail addresses, 132, 133
emotional pain, xvi, 17, 44
    and Twelve Step programs, 27–28, 34–35
essential hypertension. *See* primary hypertension
estrogen, 92
ethnic groups, 5, 6, 8–9
exercise, 5, 16, 54, 71–74, 99–116
    benefits of, 71, 109–10
    for blood circulation, 128–30
    breathing, 77–78
    for children, 10
    circuit training as, 114
    duration of, 103–4, 115
    flexibility, 100–101, 111–12
    frequency of, 103, 115
    guidelines for, 72–73, 104
    heart rate during, 103–9
    intensity of, 102, 104–5
    isotonic/isometric, 113
    as lifelong commitment, 110
    as primary treatment strategy, 99–100
    pulse rate in, 106, 109
    relaxation, 77–79, 112, 128–30
    research on, 102, 110, 112
    and stress, 76
    stretching, 111–12
    talk test during, 104
    using imagery, 127

using large muscles,
102
for weight loss, 111
with weights, 112–14
yoga, 128–30
eyes, 18, 94

F

family members, 30, 35,
40, 42–43, 45
fatigue, 11, 107
fats, 3, 5, 18, 56, 66–67,
70
in meat, 58, 59
fear, xx, 34, 41
fetal death, 93
Fifth Step, xxi, xxiii,
32–36, 37
First Step, xxi, xxii,
24–25, 28, 36
fitness, 100–105
flexibility exercises,
100–101, 112
food choices, 57–70
forgiveness, 33, 34
Fourth Step, xxi, xxii,
30–32, 33, 36, 37

Framingham Heart
Study, 132
friends, 35, 40, 42–43,
45, 49
fruits, 5, 58, 59–60, 66,
70

G

gender factors, 9, 91–97
genetic factors, 5, 9, 10,
14
ginseng, 118
God. *See* Higher Power
guilt, 34, 40, 41, 42

H

Harvard Medical School,
17–18, 88–89
HDL cholesterol, 56, 71
headaches, 11
headstands, 130
heart attacks, 3–4, 19,
96, 97
heart diseases, ix, 1, 19,
96–97
and exercise, 71
and smoking, 79

heart rates, 2, 76, 77, 80
  and biofeedback, 126
  during exercise,
    103–9
  medication for lower-
    ing, 86–87
hearts, ix, 1, 2–3, 11,
  18–19
  and alcohol consump-
    tion, 56–57
  enlarged, 4, 19
  palpitation of, 11, 73
herbal medicines, 118
high blood pressure. *See*
  hypertension
Higher Power, viii,
  xvi–xvii, 47–48, 51,
  57, 88, 116
  acceptance of, 22
  communicating with,
    29, 34, 38–39,
    45–48, 53–54
  cooperating with,
    28–29, 46, 53, 89,
    117
  and Step Two, 25–26,
    37

and Step Three,
    28–29, 37
  and Step Five, 32–34
  and Step Six, 37
  and Step Seven,
    38–39, 99
  and Step Ten, 44–45
  and Step Eleven,
    45–46
  and Step Twelve,
    48–51
  support groups as,
    26
Hispanic women, 91,
  92–93
honesty, 31–35, 37, 43
hope, 24, 25–26, 48–50
Horizontal Healer, 129
hormones, 7, 92
humility, 33, 37, 38–39,
  43
Huxley, Aldous, xviii
hypertension, ix–x, 1–2,
  10, 115–16
  alternative/comple-
    mentary treatments
    for, 117, 125–30

candidates for, 5–6,
    8–9
in children, 9–10
consequences of, 3–4,
    18–19
diagnosing, 12–15
diastolic pressure in,
    3, 11, 12, 13
as incurable disease,
    xvii, 1, 2, 16, 24
information resources
    for, 120, 131–33
pregnancy-induced,
    93–94
primary, 5, 9–10, 16,
    55–56, 75, 99–100,
    109
renovascular, 7
secondary, 7, 10, 100,
    109
stages of, 11–12
symptoms of, ix, x, 2,
    10–11, 18, 30, 84
systolic pressure in,
    2–3, 11, 12, 13
Twelve Step program

for, xxi–xxii,
    24–51, 53
white coat, 7–8, 12
See also diet; exer-
    cise; medica-
    tions; research;
    smoking
hypnosis, 126

I
idiopathic hypertension.
    See primary
    hypertension
imagery, 126–27
Index Medicus, 123
Internet, 80, 119–20,
    121, 123–24
isolation, xii, 35
isotonic/isometric exer-
    cises, 113

K
kidney problems, ix, 1, 4,
    7, 19, 85
in children, 10, 94
Knee Squeeze, 128–30

L

laboratory tests, 15, 94
laziness, 99
lifestyle changes, 57,
    81–82
loneliness, xii, 35
lungs, 4, 100–101
    cancer of, 81, 96–97

M

massage therapy, 121,
    125
meat consumption,
    58–59, 61, 63, 70
medical insurance, 117,
    125
medications, 54, 55,
    56–57, 69, 81–88
    birth control pills, 7,
        16
    for children, 10
    during pregnancy,
        94
    research on, 84, 95, 96
    side effects of, 83, 92,
        99–100

and smoking, 79
types of, 85–88
meditation, 29, 45–48,
    53, 77
    benefits of, 17–18, 46,
        88–89, 127, 128
    concentrative, 78
    as mind-body therapy,
        xv–xvi, 126
    mindfulness, 78–79
men, 9, 91, 96
menopause, 92
Mind/Body Medical
    Institute, xv, 17–18
mind-body therapies,
    17–18, 88–89, 125–30
muscle strength,
    100–101, 111, 115
muscle tension, 77, 126
music therapy, 126

N

National Heart, Lung,
    and Blood Institute
    (NHLBI), 131–32,
    133

National Institutes of
Health (NIH), xv, 118
as resource center,
120, 123, 131
nervous system in-
hibitors, 87
Nicotine Anonymous
(NA), 80
nicotine cessation strate-
gies, 79–80, 118
Ninth Step, xxi, xxiii,
42–44
NLM (U.S. National
Library of Medicine),
123
nosebleeds, 11

O
Office of Alternative
Medicine (OAM),
118–19
overweight people, 10,
68–69
and hypertension
risks, 5, 57, 68,
111

P
personal inventories,
30–32, 36, 44
physical activity. *See*
exercise
physical examinations,
13–15, 94
Power Greater. *See*
Higher Power
powerlessness, 24–25,
28, 37
practitioners, health care,
121–25
credentials of, 121,
124
locating, 121–22
prayer, 29, 34, 38–39,
45–48, 53–54
benefits of, 17–18, 46,
76, 88–89, 127
as mind-body therapy,
xv–xvi, 126
preeclampsia, 93–94
pregnancy, 93–95
prescriptions. *See*
medications

pride, 30, 38
primary hypertension, 5, 9–10, 16
  and alcohol consumption, 55–56
  and exercise, 99–100, 110
  and stress, 75
progress, 23, 39, 42, 44, 51
psychotherapy, 126
pulse rate, 106, 109

R
race factors, 5, 8–9, 10
  and gender factors, 91, 92–93, 97
relaxation exercises, 77–79, 112, 128–30
relaxation response, 76, 77
religion, viii, 26, 29–30
renal disorders, 7, 110
renin, 95
renovascular hypertension, 7

research, 124, 131–32
  on complementary/alternative therapies, 118, 119
  on exercise, 102, 110, 112
  on hypertension, 17–18, 96, 127, 128
  on medication, 84, 95, 96
  on mind-body interactions, 88–89, 125–26
  on preeclampsia, 93–94
  on smoking cessation, 79–80, 81
resentments, 41–42, 45
retinal disease, 14

S
Saint-John's-wort, 118
salt, 5, 10, 57, 58, 60–68, 85–86
saturated fats, 58, 62, 63

secondary hypertension, 7, 10, 100, 110

Second Step, xxi, xxii, 25–27, 28, 37

self-assessment. *See* personal inventories

self-awareness, 31–32, 38

self-centeredness, 22, 30

selfishness, 30, 37

self-pity, xx, 30, 44–45

self-respect, 43, 44

self-worth, 38

serenity, 23, 25, 44, 45, 53
    prayer for, 29, 39, 76

Seventh Step, xxi, xxiii, 38–39, 45, 99

sex factors, 9, 91–92

shame, 32, 34

shortcomings, 38–39, 45

shortness of breath, 11, 73

Sixth Step, xxi, xxiii, 36–38, 39

smoking, 1, 16, 40, 79
    and birth control pills, 95, 96
    and blood pressure readings, 13
    cessation of, 54, 79–81, 118
    research on, 79–80, 81

snacks, 62, 67, 70

sodium. *See* salt

sphygmomanometer, 8

spiritual awakening, 48, 50–51

spirituality, xii, 16–18, 25, 29–30
    health benefits from, vii–ix, xv–xvii, 88–89

steroids, 7, 112

strength training, 101, 112–15

stress, xv–xvi, 1, 55, 75–77, 118

stretching exercises, 111–12

strokes, 1, 3, 18, 96, 97
  types of, 4
substance abuse, vii, viii,
  xix, 55–56, 128
  and hypertension, 16,
  75
support groups, 45, 49
  as Higher Power,
  26
  as mind-body therapy,
  126
  for smoking cessation,
  80
  for Step Seven, 39
systolic pressure, 2–3,
  11, 12, 13

T
tension, 128–30
Tenth Step, xxii, xxiii,
  36, 44–45
Third Step, xxi, xxii,
  27–30, 37
Twelfth Step, xxii, xxiii,
  48–51
Twelve Step programs,

xi, xvi–xx, 21–24, 42,
  51
  for alcoholics, vii,
  xxii–xxiii
  for chronic illness,
  xii–xiii, 89, 127
  for hypertension,
  xxi–xxii, 24–51, 53
  misunderstanding of,
  xviii
  for smoking cessation,
  80
  spirituality in, 21–22,
  25–26, 50–51

U
U.S. National Library of
  Medicine (NLM), 123

V
vasodilators, 87
vegetables, 5, 58, 59–60,
  61, 64–65, 70

W
walking, 71, 72, 105–9

water pills, 85–86
Web sites, 80, 120, 132, 133
weight loss, 10, 16, 54, 69–71, 101, 111
weight training, 112–14
white-coat hypertension, 7–8, 12
Wilson, Bill, ix
women, 9, 91–97
    Asian, 93
    and birth control
    medication, 7, 16, 92, 94–95
    black, 91, 92–93, 97
    and cardiovascular diseases, 96–97
    and pregnancy-induced hyper-tension, 93–94
World Wide Web. *See* Internet; Web sites

Y
yoga, 125, 128–30

About the Author

MARK JENKINS is the author of several books on health. He co-wrote *The Sports Medicine Bible,* a Book-of-the-Month Club alternate selection. Mark lives year-round on Martha's Vineyard off the coast of Cape Cod, Massachusetts. He travels occasionally to the mainland by ferryboat to fulfill his duties as publishing consultant at the world-renowned Boston Children's Hospital.

HAZELDEN INFORMATION AND EDUCATIONAL SERVICES is a division of the Hazelden Foundation, a not-for-profit organization. Since 1949, Hazelden has been a leader in promoting the dignity and treatment of people afflicted with the disease of chemical dependency.

The mission of the foundation is to improve the quality of life for individuals, families, and communities by providing a national continuum of information, education, and recovery services that are widely accessible; to advance the field through research and training; and to improve our quality and effectiveness through continuous improvement and innovation.

Stemming from that, the mission of this division is to provide quality information and support to people wherever they may be in their personal journey—from education and early intervention, through treatment and recovery, to personal and spiritual growth.

Although our treatment programs do not necessarily use everything Hazelden publishes, our bibliotherapeutic materials support our mission and the Twelve Step philosophy upon which it is based. We encourage your comments and feedback.

The headquarters of the Hazelden Foundation is in Center City, Minnesota. Additional treatment facilities are located in Chicago, Illinois; New York, New York; Plymouth, Minnesota; St. Paul, Minnesota; and West Palm Beach, Florida. At these sites, we provide a continuum of care for men and women of all ages. Our Plymouth facility is designed specifically for youth and families.

For more information on Hazelden, please call **1-800-257-7800.** Or you may access our World Wide Web site on the Internet at **www.hazelden.org.**

Other titles that may interest you . . .